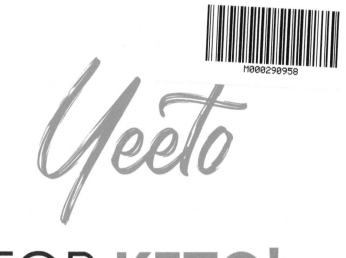

Yeeto
FOR KETO!

A Ketogenic Diet & Intermittent Fasting Experience:
Lose Weight, Burn Fat, and Live a Low-Carb Lifestyle Every Day!

TONY SCOTT & STEPHEN REZZA

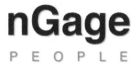

nGage
PEOPLE

Paperback ISBN: 978-0-9815545-1-8

eBook ISBN: 978-0-9815545-2-5

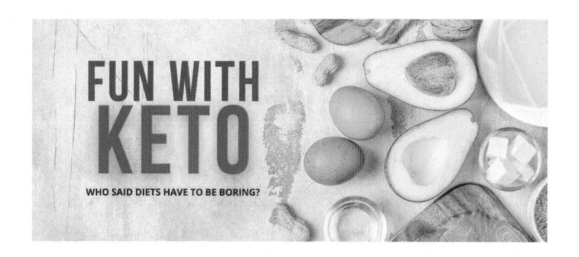

JOIN OUR FACEBOOK GROUP!

Find your tribe at **FUN WITH KETO!** A positive community focused on keeping your diet fun as you pursue a lifestyle change with the ketogenic diet. Here you will find sharing of personal success stories, keto hacks, the latest diet updates, tips, new ideas, and delicious quick-prep recipes shared by our moderators and members. Keto is more fun when you surround yourself with community. Scan the QR code below:

www.facebook.com/groups/funwithketo

HOW CAN

YOU WIN

IF

YOU NEVER

BEGIN

CONTENTS

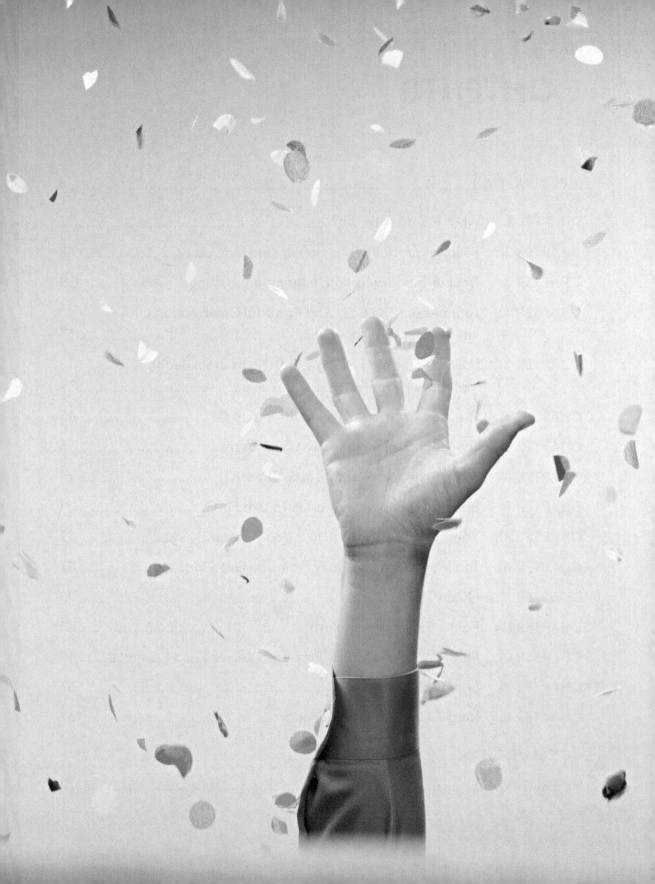

INTRODUCTION

First things first: Say "Yeet!" to a new you.

The slang word "yeet" has featured in the colloquial language for over two decades now, but its usage and popularity have changed over the years. A few years ago, a kid's video went viral on social media. His celebratory dance move with flailing hands caught people's fancy. And for reasons best known to the young minds, it was called "Yeet." Probably, it was their way of exclaiming "Yes!" which was then converted to "Yaas!" between many youngsters and finally ended up as the more energized and unique sounding "Yeet!"

It soon became a regular feature in memes. Since it began to be used in different ways and contexts, everybody was confused about the real meaning of the word.

Yeet is essentially a verb meaning to throw something away energetically with a lot of force. Following that action, you then yell, "Yeet!" as a strong emotional expression, which mostly ends up adding a humorous touch to the scene. Some people believe that the word was popularized originally by basketball players who gave a loud and guttural "Yeet!" when shooting for a slam dunk. The habit then trickled into the online gaming community lingo. The exclamation was often used by a gamer while throwing things around in frustration upon losing. Ever since, yeet has faded in and out of popular culture.

If you ask me, I like the word yeet because it sounds much like shouting out "EAT!" That's more like a blessing when the whole world is continuously hammering DIET into your head. These are diets that threaten to starve you; diets that will make a yo-yo out of your mental and physical health; and above all, diets that are so boring that you just cannot stick with them for too long.

What would you say if I were to show you a fun and effective way to lose weight? A diet that will see you "throwing" your excess weight off with ease—just like yeet is defined as the discarding of an unwanted item with velocity ("Urban Dictionary: Yeet," 2019). I am excited to share a diet plan that won't cause you to stress yourself out. A diet that won't feel like a punishment or a death sentence—a diet that will let you eat. I can almost hear you saying, "Amen!" to that right now, but I would like to coin a new way of responding here. How about "Yeeto"?

Say "Yeeto!" to Fun Diets—Forget the Old and Boring

This book is inspired by the slang word yeet, which, as you know by now, is an exclamation of excitement, approval, and all-around energy. You only wish you could gear up to lose all your excess weight with the same spirit. It could be as easy as shedding it all while maybe dabbing or flossing.

When does any aspect of our life begin to feel like a task? Whether at work, in sports, or even while traveling, getting from point A to point B will feel stressful if you are not having fun doing it. When the journey is not simple and easy to follow through, you begin to question why you started out at all. You lose motivation and interest, without which you will not get very far—let alone reach your goal.

I am sure you know at least one person who signed up for a diet program, or maybe you spent some steep money on a plan yourself that you never followed because it was terribly tedious, too complicated, or just way too much and over the top. Strict diets are hard to keep up with and sap the life out of you. After embarking upon the diet plan, you realize that it is anything but fun. The lack of creativity in the prescribed food choices by the age-old and strict diet plans can even have a contrary effect on you. Most people run the risk of binge eating out of boredom and sadly end up putting on more weight. This makes you feel that living with the status quo would have been far better. You end up regretting having started out with the diet at all.

The health food and fitness industry has conditioned you to believe that you must sacrifice many things dear to you if you wish for weight loss and good health. The traditional approach toward weight loss has always been about going on a diet that forces you to say "No." It is a NO to your social life, NO to all the happiness that good food can bring, and an even bigger NO to a natural, healthy lifestyle. Such a negative approach from the get-go! How could anyone expect a positive outcome from that?

I do know of some strict rule-oriented and extremely restrictive weight-loss regimens that give almost instant results, but arguably, I haven't come across a single soul who has been able to continue with them for more than, at a maximum, a couple of years. Weight loss achieved from a diet that is not sustainable can never be a long-lasting venture. Strict diets or diets that crash your weight drastically over a short time do not work in the long run, and we all know that now.

A scientist at the National Institutes of Health, Kevin Hall, watched the popular reality TV show, *The Biggest Loser*. He saw that each contestant lost an average of 127 pounds and nearly 64% body fat during the season. From the research conducted later, Hall learned that the phenomenal results were achieved with the help of tough trainers and doctors, strict meal plans, and killer workouts. However, he concluded that the human body fights to regain all the fat in the long run, despite all efforts. Hall observed that after a period, 13 of the 14 contestants gained back nearly 66% of the weight they had lost on the show, and four contestants had unfortunately become heavier than they were *before* the show (Sifferlin, 2017).

Dieting has to be more than just about cutting calories. It must be more focused on bringing about a gradual and steady transformation. Your diet has to be about eating food that tastes good, makes you feel good, and makes you feel full. For weight loss to be sustainable, the diet needs to be easy to incorporate into your daily life. It cannot be a quick-fix idea. You should find it becoming a habit. I believe we can all adapt to a healthy and balanced lifestyle without draining all the cheer out of our life.

Say "Yeeto!" to eating joyfully and having fun while working toward weight loss and aiming to burn fat. Forget the old and boring weight-loss diet ideas.

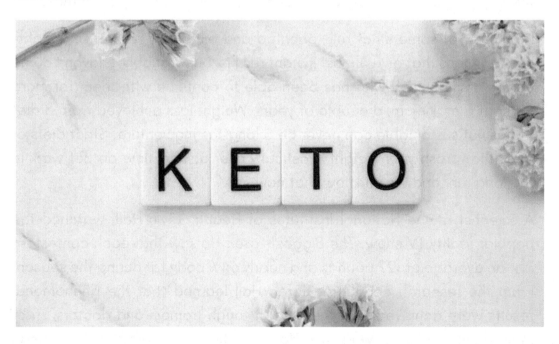

Yeeto for Keto! is written in an intentionally casual tone. I wish to speak with you and not at you. You should have as much fun following this diet plan as I had while writing it for you. I wish you to see how the ketogenic diet combined with intermittent fasting can be an effective and fun way to lose weight while also guaranteeing fabulous results.

The sections in this book have been carefully planned to guide you throughout your diet journey. You will find detailed explanations of why combining the ketogenic diet with intermittent fasting will prove to be a great weight-loss and fat-burning strategy, as well as specifics about how to smoothly adapt to the lifestyle change. This book has some keto-friendly, quick, easy-to-prepare, and surprisingly delicious recipes. You can keep both your taste buds and tummy happy with a healthy supply of good food. Before you proceed to the keto hacks and fun facts sections, there are some tips and recommendations on how you can track your success daily.

However, you must keep in mind that there are two rules of thumb for successful weight loss and fat burning. Your diet plan and strategy are unique to you. Understand and observe what works best for you as an individual. Don't follow the crowd mentality. Take note of how your metabolism uniquely responds to the diet plan. And finally, you will come to realize that the strategy is only effective for burning fat and weight loss when followed consistently.

To quote Confucius, "It does not matter how slowly you go, as long as you don't stop" (quotespedia.org, n.d.).

His words may not originally have been for those aspiring to weight loss, but it sure does sound like great advice. Lastly, don't make it a competition. Enjoy the process. When you begin to see results, say yeet for a new you!

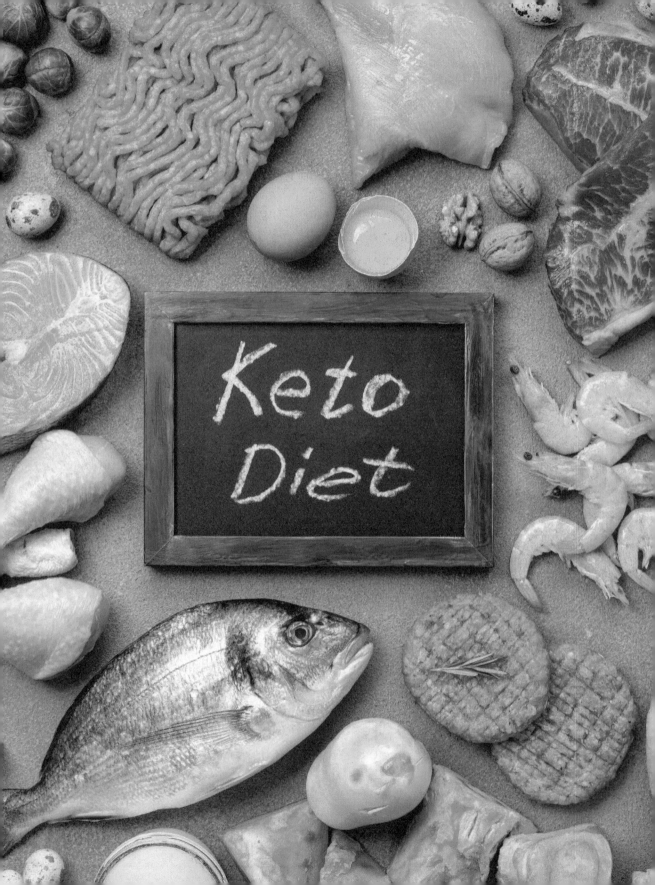

Chapter 1:
What is Keto After All?

The ketogenic diet, the hero of this book, is your friend, so feel free to nickname it keto. You must acquaint yourself with everything that keto is all about before you set out on your journey with the diet. You will automatically see why you need keto if you understand how the keto diet works for your body.

The number-one supply of energy for your body comes from carbohydrates. When you eat food made up of carbohydrates, it is converted into glucose, or blood sugar, which energizes the cells in your body. The ketogenic diet is primarily based on the principle that, by depriving your body of carbohydrates, you push your body to burn fats for fuel, thereby maximizing weight loss. The ketogenic diet is, therefore, a high-fat, low-carb, and only adequate protein diet plan.

What Is Ketosis?

When you replace the carbs in your diet with fats, your body is sent into the metabolic state of ketosis. In this process, due to the limited supply of glucose due to the absence of carbs, fats get broken down in the liver to produce ketone bodies. The ketones produced are then used as an alternative source to derive energy for your cells. The fun bit about breaking down fat as your energy resource is that you will feel satiated for a longer time. The high-fat content of the diet is responsible for the increase in the production of the hormone called leptin, which suppresses your appetite. Not feeling hungry while your body is losing weight is obviously advantageous.

On the other hand, ghrelin—the hunger hormone that is mainly produced in the stomach—is responsible for stimulating the appetite. The ketogenic diet reduces the secretion of ghrelin and thus prevents the urge for more food.

Scientific research has confirmed the hunger-reduction phenomenon reported during ketogenic diets. Body-weight regulation is controlled by two important mechanisms: hunger and satiety. Even though we think we can control our eating by will, our central nervous system (CNS) regulates our food intake and energy expenditure more than we can imagine. The control center is spread over different brain areas which receive information from the adipose tissue, gastrointestinal tract (GIT), and blood and peripheral sensory receptors. The hunger and satiety signals from the brain are influenced by nutrients, hormones, and other signaling molecules. Ketone bodies become the energy source in times of carbohydrate shortage and influence food intake control (Paoli et al., 2015).

Don't forget to note that if you supply your body with more protein than it needs, your body will convert the extra protein into glucose. This is called gluconeogenesis which can hamper your weight loss. That's why you must consciously consume proper proportions of fat, carbs, and protein to keep your weight-loss program on track.

Often people confuse the low-carb diet with the ketogenic diet. The difference lies in the macros that keto prioritizes and the intake ratio for the macros. Also, there are several types of ketogenic diets based on different theories and research. But let us focus on the standard keto and get our keto basics right. The typically recommended intake ratio is 70% fat, 25% protein, and only a nominal amount of 5% carbs.

In the words of Kristen Kizer, a registered clinical dietician at Houston Methodist Hospital in Texas, "A keto diet to me would be any diet that gets a body into ketosis" (Lawler, 2020).

Why Follow Keto?

Keto has become an increasingly popular weight-loss strategy over the past few years for individuals who are overweight as well as those who are health-conscious in everyday situations. Social media has been instrumental in spreading the word, but this diet has been around for quite a long time and it has been known to provide many more health benefits beyond just weight loss.

In 1921, Dr. Russel Wilder from the Mayo Clinic first used a high-fat diet to treat epilepsy. He suggested that the high-fat diet would result in ketonemia that would reduce seizures. Dr. Wilder coined the title the "Ketogenic Diet" (KD). In the medical world, KD, the ketone-producing diet, became immensely favored as a therapeutic diet for pediatric epilepsy (Kim, 2017).

However, a lesser-known fact is that there is a low-carb, high-fat predecessor to KD. The successful application of the diet for weight loss is attributed to a 19th century retired funeral director named William Banting. A physician from Soho Square named William Harvey had learned about a diet plan for diabetes management. Essentially, it is slightly different from the ketogenic diet we know. Dr. Harvey prescribed the plan to Banting, who followed it and successfully reduced his weight by nearly 50 pounds. In 1863, Banting self-published an open letter and described how obesity was the cause of degeneration, illness, and health-related evils. Banting triggered a phenomenon in the Victorian era. Slimness became the marker of privilege and prestige, but more importantly, the English were sensitized to the hazards of obesity.

Today, the medical world is far more advanced—new innovations are being made constantly—yet obesity continues to remain a terrifying global health hazard. Adult mortality due to obesity has been recorded at 2.8 million per year. It is sad to observe that those suffering from obesity develop chronic diseases like diabetes, hypertension, and heart disease. An unhealthy lifestyle and poor dietary habits have been identified as the root causes of this evil. An appropriate and personalized diet plan for weight loss can offer a solution for obesity. Thankfully, scientific research has busted the misconceptions and proven that the low-carbohydrate and the high-fat ketogenic diet is very effective for rapid weight loss (Masood & Uppaluri, 2019).

Though the ketogenic diet was created as a part of the treatment for epilepsy, it has progressively proven to have multiple benefits for a wide range of medical issues. Therefore, following keto can work wonders as a preventive or precautionary measure for metabolic, neurological, or insulin-related problems, too.

When you eat, the pancreas releases the hormone called insulin. The primary role of insulin is to help our organs with the assimilation of blood glucose. When there is an excess of blood sugar levels, the organs stop responding to insulin. This is called insulin resistance, which causes the glucose to get deposited in your bloodstream. The continued state of excess sugar in the blood can, unfortunately, lead you to enter the prediabetes stage. If blood sugar levels stay high over a long period, it causes high blood pressure. Insulin resistance can lead to fatty liver disease, polycystic ovary syndrome (PCOS), and heart conditions.

Keto restricts the supply of carbohydrates which would have caused the blood sugar levels to spike in your body with all the glucose produced. By controlling blood glucose levels, keto alleviates insulin resistance and regulates blood pressure. This is a direct benefit to those suffering from prediabetes, type 2 diabetes, and heart conditions. Improved insulin sensitivity can also help reduce PCOS.

Nearly 90% of adolescents and teens suffer from acne that persists into adulthood. In Western countries, around 50% of people in their 20s and 30s struggle with acne. About 15 years of extensive research has confirmed that refined carbohydrates may be the dietary culprit causing acne due to their negative effects on hormonal regulation. Ketogenic diet plans that cut carbs are known to reduce insulin resistance and have anti-inflammatory effects. Thus, keto proves to be therapeutic as it controls inflammation which drives acne progression (Spritzler, 2021).

Since the ketogenic diet helps burn body fat, it lowers the low-density lipoprotein (LDL), or bad cholesterol levels, and triglycerides, thus considerably reducing the risk of developing cardiovascular diseases. Regulated blood pressure and cholesterol help to improve heart health.

The ketogenic diet has a significant neuroprotective impact on the brain. When ketones replace carbs as an energy source, there is an increase in the production of neurotransmitters. They act as the chemical messengers responsible for transmitting information from one nerve cell to another. Thus, there is more efficient communication between neurons in the brain leading to improved brain function.

Since the ketogenic diet reduces dependency on glucose for energy metabolism, it considerably increases resistance to metabolic stress and resilience to neuronal loss. There is some scientific evidence of the effectiveness of the ketogenic diet in treating central nervous system injuries or disorders such as epilepsy, hypoxia, and ischemic stroke. The keto diet is key to the successful treatment of neurodegenerative disorders, like amyotrophic lateral sclerosis (ALS), Addison's disease (AD), and Parkinson's disease (Erdman et al., 2011).

A report published in the journal *Cell Reports* suggested that restricting your blood sugar helps to combat certain cancerous tumor growths, as reported by Dr. William Li:

> Ketogenic diets are known to interfere with tumor growth in more ways than one ... [The diet] triggers a chain reaction of at least three other cancer-fighting mechanisms ... Ketogenic diets also lower the tumor's [growth] ... by cutting off the tumor blood supply ... [and the] cancer cells become starved and can't grow (Holland, 2019, para. 4).

Additionally, keto helps increase cell sensitivity to treatments like chemotherapy and radiation. However, it is always advisable to consult a registered dietician who specializes in oncology nutrition to check that the patient is able to maintain the keto diet and stay healthy (Holland, 2019).

Short-Term Side Effects of Keto

Switching from the usual carbohydrates to fats as your energy source is a massive change for your body. It should be expected that your body will take time to accept it. While the body is adjusting, you might experience some short-term side effects like headaches, vomiting, gastrointestinal discomfort, loose movements, and fatigue during the initial phase. Sometimes, the string of bad symptoms may make you feel like you have the flu, and that's why it is called the keto flu or the low-carb flu.

Some experts might caution you of another common side effect: hypoglycemia. Breaking into a sweat or chills, excessive thirst, increased frequency of urination, and light-headedness are some of the signs to watch out for.

You may begin to worry and even consider quitting due to the side effects. However, you must remind yourself that this is just a temporary phase. If you bear with it and continue with the keto diet until your body has adjusted properly, you will begin to experience the benefits of the diet, too. You can also drink a lot of water to reduce the severity of the side effects.

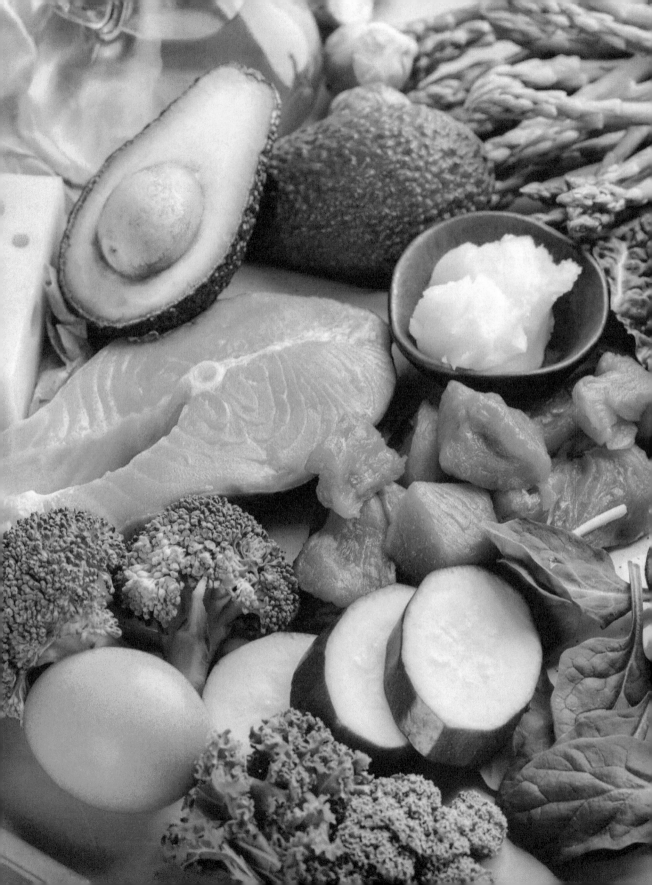

Chapter 2:
Following a Daily Formula for Keto Macros

Good health and balanced nutrition are what keep us fit and fine to shoot a hoop, hula-hoop, tango, or exert our energy in any other way we like. You may want to know more about

"Food is our body's fuel," says Rebecca Solomon, director of clinical nutrition in New York City. "If we don't use high-grade fuel, we can't expect high functioning"

(Bowers, 2014).

nutrients while learning about the ketogenic diet. Whatever you eat or drink is constantly supplying your body with nutrients. The correct diet will give you the right amount of nutrients needed for healthy metabolic activities and to improve and maintain good health or protect yourself from or fight diseases.

Nutrition for our body is acquired in two nutrient groups: the macronutrients and the micronutrients. Carbohydrates, fats, and proteins are the macronutrients that are required in large quantities. Vitamins and minerals are the micronutrients needed in relatively small amounts.

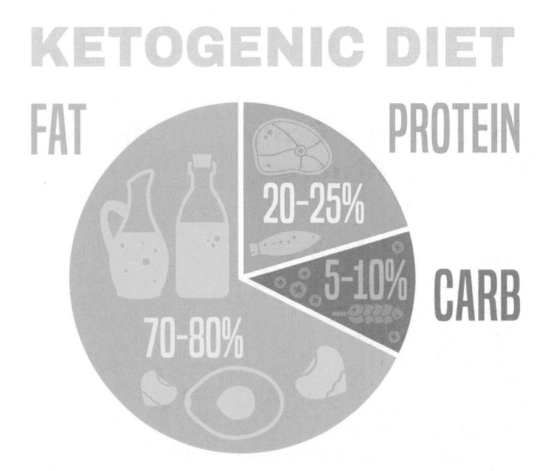

Know Your Macros

Macros are the primary source of energy for our body and mind to function smoothly. Some macros become more essential to our body at particular stages in life or are required by specific age groups or people suffering from malnutrition or disease.

Carbohydrates

Carbs are arguably the most favorite macros in any part of the world, and that is why you must understand what a carbohydrate is to fully grasp its role as a macronutrient.

Our body turns to carbohydrates as its favored source of energy. Carbs are broken down into blood sugar or glucose that powers our metabolism and brain functions. However, did you know that there are two types of carbohydrates? Simple carbohydrates are known as the source of bad carbs, and complex carbohydrates give us good carbs. The chemical composition of the carbs we eat and the time our body takes to digest the food will tell you if you have just eaten a complex carb or a simple carb.

Who doesn't salivate at the thought of sugary sweets and starchy foods? Loaves of bread, pasta, sweetened yogurt, and cereals are just a few of the foods you devour that are categorized as refined or processed carbohydrates. It is sad but true that most packaged foods contribute massive amounts of bad carbs to your diet. Our body immediately breaks down the bad carbs to make sugar, which causes our blood glucose levels to unhealthily rise and fall quickly.

This macronutrient is also found in fibrous foods, which are known as complex carbohydrates. Save for a few starchy vegetables and fruits, plant-based fresh foods are rich in fiber and give us mostly good carbs. Whole foods like beans, nuts, and grains are a good source of carbohydrates. Our body breaks down the complex carbs very slowly, and that's why they won't cause a spike in blood sugar levels. Also, complex carbohydrates contain small traces of vitamins and minerals needed for our body.

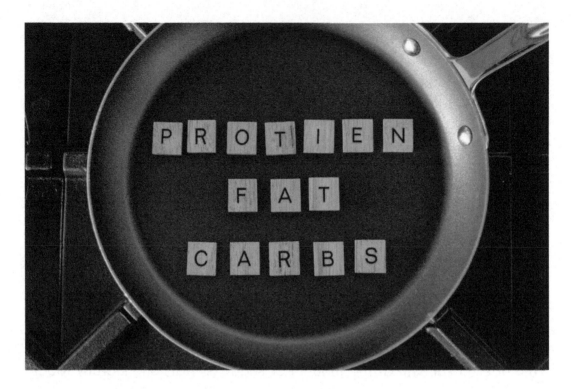

Proteins

One can safely say that people all over the world are obsessed with protein mania. You simply cannot blame them because protein is indeed a vital macronutrient for our body. Each and every cell and muscle in our body needs these organic compounds.

Proteins are made up of innumerable little building blocks called amino acids which catalyze the biochemical reactions in our body. Proteins are needed to produce enzymes, generate antibodies that protect us from viruses and bacteria, for the repair and recovery of body tissues from wear and tear; and to synthesize growth hormones and neurotransmitters.

Yet our body does not store proteins, so you will need to refill your protein stocks regularly. Also, try and eat a wide variety of healthy protein sources like legumes, nuts, seeds, whole grains, fresh fish, poultry, and eggs. It is the source of the protein that matters more than the consumption in large quantities.

Fats

We all consume fats, but do you know how this third essential macronutrient works for our body? Even though the oldest myth that fats are fattening has been busted, the macronutrient is still considered something that should be limited in our daily diet. Like a true hero, keto has helped to turn this macro into a winner over the past few years.

The macro provides us with essential fatty acids that are not produced in our body but need to be obtained from the foods we eat. Fat helps our nervous system function properly, helps keep us warm, and provides insulation for particular organs. Fat aids in building strong bones and teeth while also cushioning our joints and protecting them against traumatic injuries. Fats assist with the absorption of fat-soluble vitamins A, D, E, and K—all needed for healthy skin and hair. Those who do not consume enough fats face various problems like acne, rough skin, dry hair, brittle nails, fatigue, depression, etc.

You can include fats in your diet by eating animal products such as meat, fish, cheese, and eggs. It is present in nuts, seeds, legumes, and vegetables. However, it would be useful to note that not all fats are equal. There are two groups of fats: the good fats are called unsaturated fats and the bad fats are known as saturated. You should opt for unsaturated fats because they come with many health benefits. The good fats improve satiety and make you feel full longer, improve blood circulation by keeping your arteries clean, improve immunity by working like antioxidants to fight free radicals, and fats can also give you healthy skin and hair.

Now you have acquainted yourself with each macro and both of its good and bad avatars. But you may have guessed by now that while following the ketogenic diet, you cannot think in black and white; you should never look at fats as good and carbohydrates as bad macros. All the macros are required for good nutrition, but the quantity of the source must be regulated. While following the ketogenic diet plan with weight loss in mind, you must count your keto macros.

If you didn't know this before, let me tell you that counting macros is an entirely different ball game from counting the calories in your foods. When you count calories, you are looking at the units of energy you get from what you have eaten. If we are talking nutrition, it can get misleading if you are only looking at the calorie count. You could very well have reached your daily target or stayed within the daily budget of calorie intake by eating junk food, too, but when you are calculating your macros, you are carefully considering the nutrients in every gram. Don't you think it's wiser and more effective to keep a keen eye on the macros within the calories?

The ketogenic diet is all about *what* you are eating!

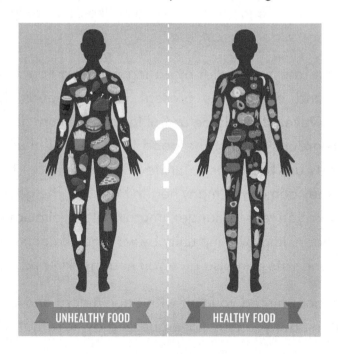

The Winning Macro Formula

I can already imagine you gearing up to win this challenge of dropping those extra pounds, so let's give our happy war cry, "Yeeto!" loud and clear for keto and burn some fat right away.

The ketogenic diet shows you how to derive the best nutrition from each macro by consuming it in the most appropriate quantities. Get your keto macros right and you will have upskilled your capability of reaching ketosis.

Even as I tell you that there is a formula for you to follow to calculate your daily keto macro intake, don't worry—you won't hear me saying, "Do the math!" I know, keeping a tab day in and day out and counting the macros in every gram you eat or drink already sounds tedious.

There are easy-to-use keto macro calculators available online that can be your go-to tool throughout your ketogenic diet journey. You can easily calculate keto macros catered for optimal results for your age, physique, gender, and daily physical activity levels. However, for simply being in the know, I will share how keto macros are calculated manually.

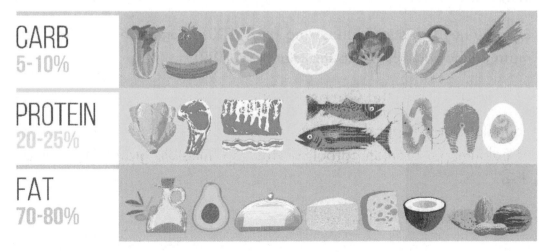

KETOGENIC DIET HIGH FAT LOW PROTEIN LOW CARB

CARB
5-10%

PROTEIN
20-25%

FAT
70-80%

Counting Your Macros

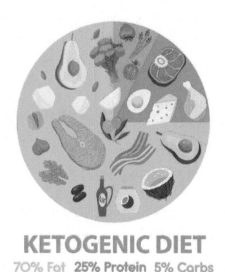

KETOGENIC DIET
70% Fat **25% Protein** 5% Carbs

There is no bigger goal than reaching ketosis by maintaining the ideal keto macro ratio in every meal. Like I mentioned before, you must take care that 70% of the calories in your meal come from fat, 25% from protein, and only 5% from carbs.

That's why you must first know that every gram of carbs contains four calories, every gram of fat has nine calories, and every gram of protein has four calories.

Knowledge is power, and math can come in very handy. If you know your daily calorie intake goal for weight loss, you could calculate the keto macros for each meal, too. Remember, you must maintain a calorie deficit in order to burn fat and lose weight. Daily calorie goals vary from person to person, depending upon your physical stats and whether you engage in exercise or not.

Say you need to stick with eating only 1,500 calories per day. Then the math will go something like this (Saunion, 2019):

Step 1: Counting the Carbs

Formula: Calories per day x percentage of calories from carbs / number of calories per gram in carbohydrates = permissible grams of carbs per day

For example, 1500 x 0.05 / 4 = 8.3

> **Pro Tip:** Your body uses only carbs to make glucose, not fiber. Since fiber has no effect on your blood glucose levels, it would be even more beneficial to eat carbs that are rich in fiber.

Step 2. Count Your Proteins

Formula: Calories per day x percentage of calories from protein / number of calories per gram in protein = permissible grams of protein per day

For example, 1500 x 0.25 / 4 = 41.6

> **Pro Tip:** You need to remember that you cannot exceed your daily allowance of 25% protein intake. Excess protein will get converted into glucose and you do not want your weight-loss plan to fail. For your body to get into ketosis and burn fat you must be sure not to supply extra protein that could be broken down for energy.

Step 3. Finally, Count Your Fat Intake

Formula: Calories per day x percentage of calories from fat / number of calories per gram in fat = grams of fat per day

For example, 1500 x 0.70 / 9 = 116.6

Counting keto macros is as simple as that!

If you count your macros and stick with the percentage distribution, all should be well in your keto life. However, it is important to consult with a doctor or your nutritionist if you have any health conditions.

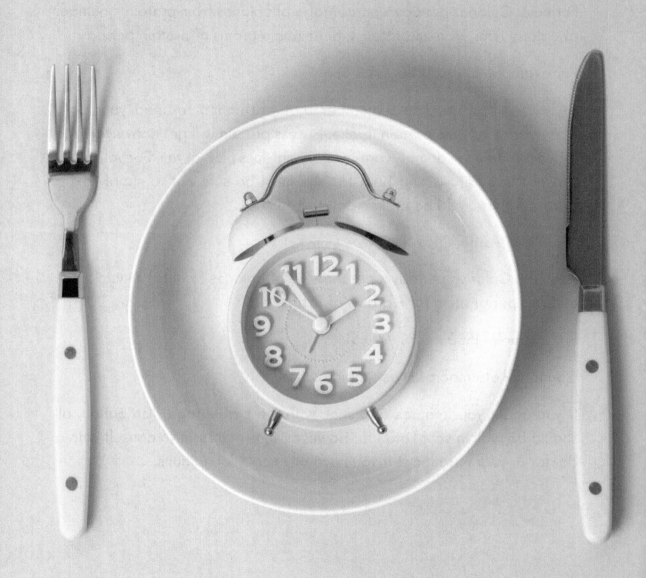

Chapter 3:

Double the Results with Intermittent Fasting — "Coolio!"

If you are cool enough to keto, then I imagine you are cool enough to adapt to any change. Intermittent fasting will change your lifestyle and will change the way you look at fasting for weight loss. Since it is the coolest fasting strategy doing the rounds, I can imagine it will be the best way to get you to your weight loss goals even quicker.

If keto has got you focusing on *what* you are eating, intermittent fasting will make you want to focus on *when* you are eating. Intermittent fasting means restricting your calorie intake to specific time slots. There will be a scheduled time for you to eat and a set time to fast. There are different intermittent fasting plans based on various combinations of fasting and eating cycles. You are free to choose the best schedule that suits your convenience and preferences.

They say the key to the success of intermittent fasting for weight loss is discipline, but whatever you do, do not make it a task. You will look back upon your weight-loss journey with a smile if you have enjoyed it at every step. When you pick the most effective fasting strategy for weight loss, ensure that you are going with something YOU like, and you will surely find it even easier to follow through.

Five Ways of Intermittent Fasting for You

You can choose from the five most popular intermittent fasting methods. Each is proven to be effective for weight loss, improving metabolism, better mental clarity, and achieving longevity, too.

1. The Time-Restricted Eating Method

You have two choices again while planning how to divide your daily hours into fasting and eating windows. You can either keep the eating window open for eight hours and fast for the remaining 16 hours, or you could eat for 10 hours and fast for the rest. In short, you have two options: 16/8 or 14/10.

The trick is to try and overlap the fasting hours with your sleeping hours. Say you have a good healthy breakfast at 9 a.m. Then, you finish eating all the meals for the day within the next eight hours and start fasting in the evening from 5 p.m. Alternatively, you could maintain a 10-hour eating window and start your fast from 7 p.m.

You do not need to limit your calorie intake, but please try and eat clean during the eating cycle. A healthy diet will give a head start to the success of your weight loss mission.

2. The 5:2 Diet Method

Some see this as a relatively challenging method. For two days of the week, you must restrict your calorie intake to only 500 calories. On your fasting days, usually two meals of 200 calories and 300 calories each are prescribed. On the remaining days of the week, you could eat as usual without any calorie restrictions. However, be sure not to plan your fasting days back-to-back. There should always be at least one eating day between the two.

Some find this method of intermittent fasting convenient because you are free to pick which two days of the week you would be fasting according to your social calendar. Your fasting would not interfere with your social life, and you are free to eat whatever you choose in the company of your friends and family.

Once again, the rule of thumb is to eat healthily and normally. No binge eating, no junk foods, and sweetened carbonated drinks are best avoided.

3. Alternate-Day Fasting Method

As per this method of intermittent fasting, you are expected to fast every alternate day. Your eating would be restricted to a 500-calorie budget or 25% of your regular intake on fasting days. On the remaining days, you could eat as much as you please.

4. The 24-Hour Fasting Method

In this method, you choose one day of the week when you will not eat at all: 24 hours of total fasting. Some also manage to do this twice a week.

The trick here is to start fasting right after a heavy breakfast or a massive lunch and continue fasting until breakfast or lunch the next day.

5. The Meal-Skipping Method

This is arguably the most popular intermittent fasting method. You decide which meal of the day you would be most okay to skip eating. General observation says that people tend to skip their breakfast because it is an activity that you need to factor in with the start of a hectic day; though starting a busy day on an empty stomach doesn't sound like a good idea either. But, then again, you could compensate by planning to have a hearty lunch and good food for the rest of the day.

The other popular choice is skipping dinner. You could easily pull it off by mentally and physically preparing yourself for it through the day. This would support the old notion that it is always better to wean off the quantity you eat by the end of the day.

One universal trick for all fasting methods is to surf those fasting hours when awake, you can drink a lot of water, coffee, and other zero-calorie beverages.

Every method of intermittent fasting mentioned has its own pros and cons. It would be best to refer to a certified physician before you make your selection and start off with any fasting plan. If you have suffered from eating disorders, are pregnant, or are breastfeeding, it isn't a good idea to start intermittent fasting. Focus on maintaining good health and practicing healthy dietary habits.

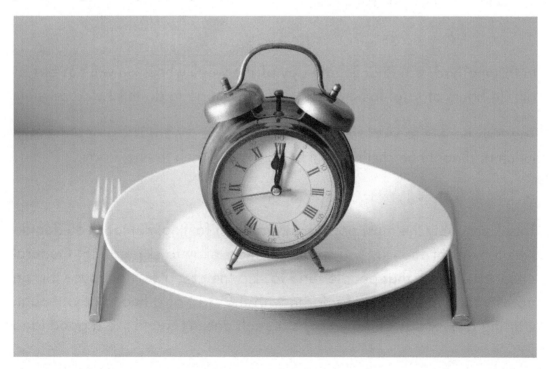

Short-Term Side Effects of Intermittent Fasting

As a force of habit, your body's immediate response to any drastic change is almost always rebellion. Be as stubborn as you can and stick with your plan. I can assure you that if the intermittent fasting plan you have chosen is right for you, and you are following the basic rules, any side effects that you may experience will only be short-lived ones.

Headaches, giddiness, and nausea can be the result of going on an empty stomach. The body will take time to adjust to the changed timelines and limited supply of food. Hunger pangs can also disrupt your sleep patterns in the initial phase. You may experience heartburn, which is caused by the rising levels of stomach acids when there is no food to process. Weakness and fatigue are common side effects when your body and mind are still learning to accept the new fasting-eating cycles. However, the most embarrassing side effect that you may notice is bad breath. When the oral cavity remains dry and empty for a long while, the acetones produced from the breaking down of fat enter your breath and release a bad odor.

These side effects are not known to have any severe impact on health, but having said that, it is always advisable that you consult a doctor if problems persist or are aggravated over a long period. If you are undergoing any medical treatment, you need to make sure that your intermittent fasting is not interrupting your medication schedule as some prescription drugs cannot be administered on an empty stomach.

Benefits of Intermittent Fasting

Modern urban populations are largely used to long periods of high-calorie eating daily coupled with a sedentary lifestyle. Obesity results from an imbalance between energy intake and energy expenditure, leading to excessive storage of spare energy as fat in the adipose tissues. The primary function of adipose tissues is to create buffer reserves of fatty acids to be broken down for energy in case of longer periods of food deprivation. Scientific research has suggested the use of intermittent fasting as a therapeutic intervention; intermittent fasting supports adipose thermogenesis for fatty acid oxidation which means intermittent fasting is a promising approach toward treating obesity (Kim et al., 2017).

Besides weight loss and fat loss, studies have confirmed that intermittent fasting can give you many other health benefits. Intermittent fasting, when followed to a T, can boost your metabolism and reduce inflammation. It can also help you prevent and fight various diseases and health conditions.

Research has proven that the 8-hour eating window helps reduce blood pressure in adults with obesity. It has been reported that intermittent fasting reduces fasting glucose by 3-6% in those with prediabetes and decreases fasting insulin by 11-57% after 3 to 24 weeks of intermittent fasting (Leonard, 2020).

Thus, it protects you from or improves type 2 diabetes, heart conditions, neurodegenerative diseases, and some cancers, too.

Although not yet scientifically proven through human testing, intermittent fasting is said to slow down aging.

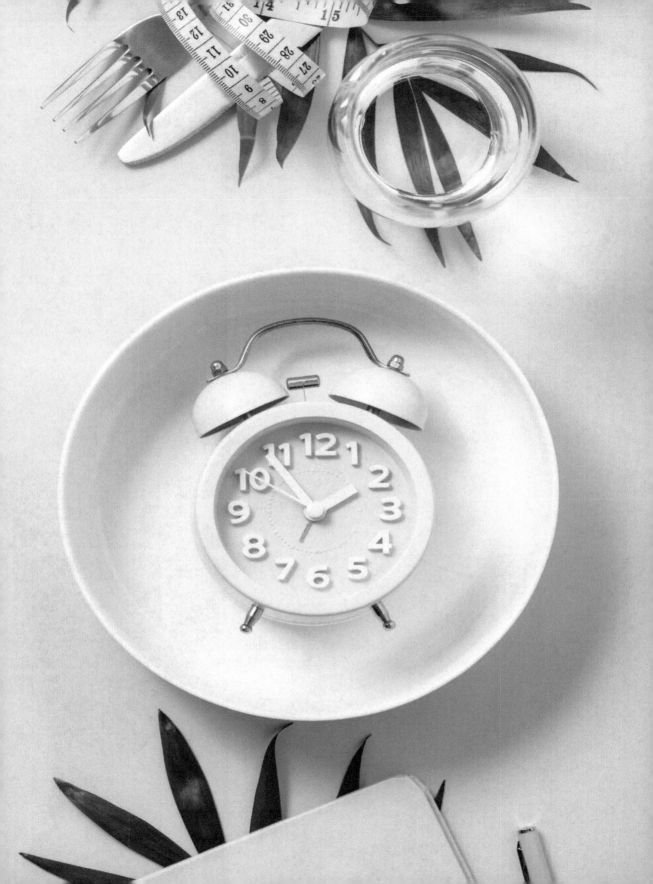

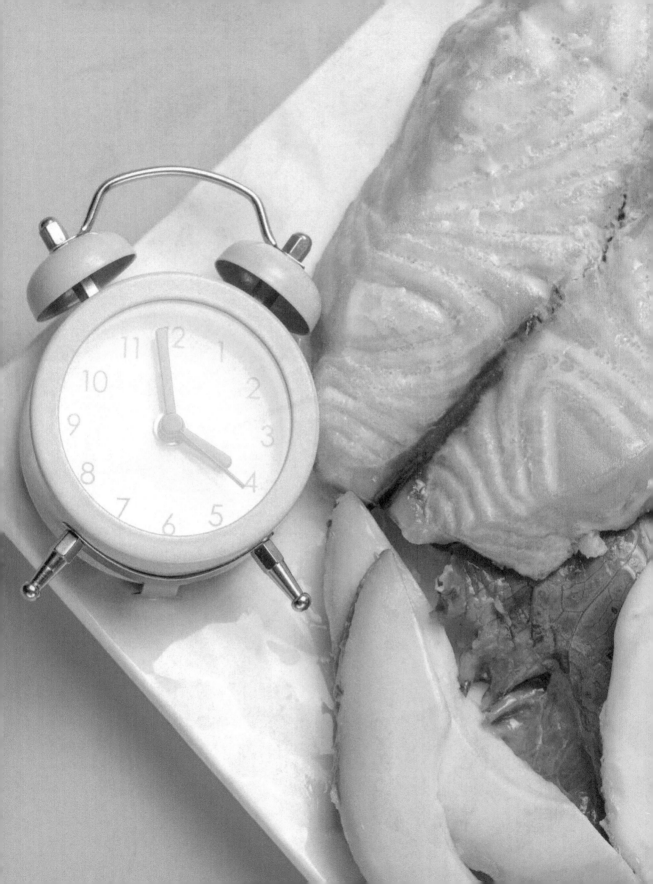

Chapter 4:

Learn about the Easy and Powerful Combination of Intermittent Fasting + Keto

One and one together make 11. No, I don't have my math wrong. What I'm giving you here is a tad philosophical—a bit more creative thinking. When one great idea is put together with another great idea, what you get is something more than your expectations.

You have set your weight loss goals, and you really want to get there. What I'm showing you is a route to get there faster. Isn't a two-wheeler faster than a unicycle? Then don't waste time overthinking things. Just get on it and get moving twice as fast.

Intermittent fasting and keto together make a fantastic combination for an effective weight-loss and healthy-living strategy. This power combo is trending because it has already given mind-blowing results and jaw-dropping transformations to many who began practicing the revolutionary intermittent keto plan.

The Power Combo

Dr. Mark Mattson, a Johns Hopkins neuroscientist, has studied intermittent fasting for 25 years. He says, "In the after-hours without food, the body exhausts its sugar stores and starts burning fat, and this is known as metabolic switching." Thus, intermittent fasting works by subjecting the body to a prolonged period when it burns through all the calories consumed in the last meal and is forced to begin burning fats for energy (John Hopkins Medicine, 2021).

That sounded much like keto, didn't it? Ketosis is also about fat oxidation for energy. Since the ketogenic diet is based on metabolic switching elicited by cutting down on carbohydrates, it is as if intermittent fasting and keto were always meant to be put together.

So if you are sticking with the keto macros formula for eating while following one of the intermittent fasting methods, you are onto something! Intermittent fasting will help you put your body into ketosis sooner. Additionally, you may find that you are burning more body fat than you did while following keto alone.

This is a strategy that practitioners counsel patients on at the Cleveland Clinic's Functional Ketogenics Program. "Adding intermittent fasting can take things up to the next level," says a certified physician at the clinic, Logan Kwasnicka. It is helpful for overcoming a weight-loss plateau, as you may eat fewer calories during intermittent fasting. Since ketosis decreases appetite, it can also feel like a natural progression from a keto diet for those who get satiated from eating so much fat and aren't bothered by shrinking their eating window (Migala, 2019).

How to Do Intermittent Keto

In every sphere of life, you need a guru to show you the way. A master—a teacher who can help you pick up a skill and even upskill gradually. Note that "gradually" is the keyword here. For any transformation in life, you need to be patient. Take it one step at a time and make steady progress until you can fully comprehend the skill.

Let me show you how to transition from one level of achievement to another gradually. Separately, both intermittent fasting and keto can be referred to as a lifestyle in their own right. When put together, you could be enjoying a pool of various health benefits brought on by each. But don't get all excited and put the cart before the horse.

Oh, I know you are not the type who would travel old style, but even if you have just hit the ignition to start on your cool and fast weight-loss journey, don't hit the pedal on the combination plan just yet.

Take it easy. Begin by slowly introducing your body to the ketogenic diet first because it is one tough, fat, cookie to crack—pun intended! Let your body take its time to adjust to the idea of burning fat for energy. You don't want to call upon the whole motherload of side effects at once by starting with intermittent fasting right now. After you feel you are getting cozy with keto, and once you are in a happier place, you could consider upgrading your weight loss to the next level. Since your body has already accepted fat oxidation as the way of life, intermittent fasting shouldn't feel like a challenge. Brigid Titgemeier, RDN, a functional medicine dietician, explains it further:

> Intermittent fasting can be paired with any kind of diet because it simply refers to the number of hours that you fast. Combining keto with intermittent fasting means adhering to the parameters of a ketogenic diet and eating within a condensed window of time
>
> (Bradley & Santilli, 2020, para. 16).

Begin by choosing the intermittent fasting method that appears relatively easy to follow at the start, or you could even take guidance from an expert on what would be most suitable for you in particular.

Thus, with intermittent keto, there are three aspects that you need to factor into your daily routine. You will need to figure it all out with a bit of time planning and learn to live with discipline from here on. Plan all your meals for the day based on how much fat and protein you are eating while restricting the carbs, when you are going to eat it, and carefully consider the quality of what you are eating. I will soon share some quick and easy-to-make keto recipes in this very book.

Intermittent fasting, when combined with keto can only boost the effect that each has on our weight loss and fat-burning mission. Gradually, you could intensify your fasting cycles while using keto recipes to plan your meals if you wish to get faster and even better results. It all depends on how your body responds to your endeavors.

If it has been a great streak then you know what you should do next. Give a loud "Yeeto!" for intermittent keto and do the happy dance.

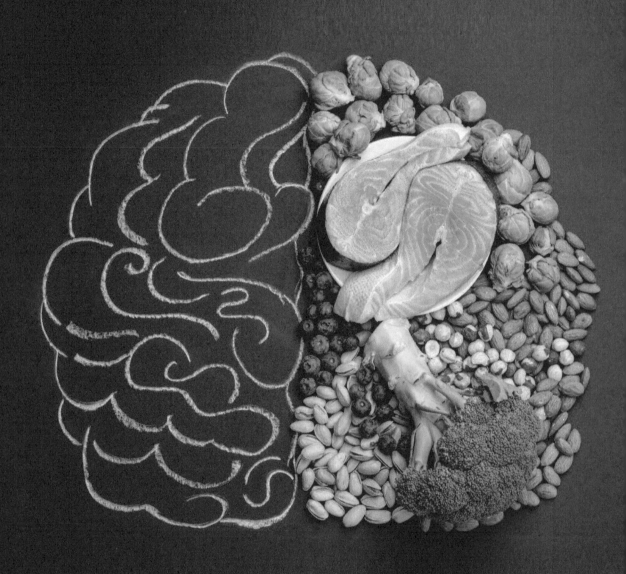

Chapter 5:

How Intermittent Fasting + Keto Helps Brain Health and Metabolism Pronto!

Stop and ponder. Here is some food for thought. We all know that the brain is arguably the most important part of our body, yet why don't we all care to give it what it really needs to stay healthy? Do we really know what brain food is to begin with?

Although the brain is only a minor percent of our body weight, at least 20% of the total calories consumed go to the brain. The brain is both the most energy-hungry and also the most energy-producing organ in your body. Your brain needs a constant supply of energy to keep it working with full gusto. The brain is also the fattiest organ—made up of 60% fat. While the connection between diet and physical health is now common knowledge, not all are aware of the role of our diet in the upkeep of our brain health. We still see physical and mental health as very separate concepts, whereas they are more interrelated than you would ever imagine (The Charlie Foundation, n.d.).

So let's get around to finding out how intermittent fasting and the ketogenic diet help improve our brain health and metabolism pronto!

Boosting Brain Health

The lack of sufficient supply of energy and blood to the brain causes most mental illnesses. If you consume a high-carb diet, you are supplying excessive amounts of glucose to your body. When the body is high on blood sugar levels, we know that blood pressure can get out of control. The increased demand for insulin to regulate blood pressure will lead to a condition called insulin insensitivity. When the body cannot handle the high blood glucose levels, it enters the prediabetic stage or develops diabetes. Diabetes can cause blood clots to block arteries which cut off the blood supply to the brain. Thus, you see, a high-carb diet can cause severe damage to the brain, from mild cognitive disorders to dementia and stroke.

Reading between the lines, we must switch the source of energy supply to our bodies and brains. Metabolizing fat instead of glucose can protect the brain from cell stress, dysfunction, and death. Contrary to popular belief that the brain can only run on glucose, research has proven that ketones can supply up to 75% of the total energy that the brain needs. The ketogenic diet gets you into ketosis, which is also known to aid the growth and efficiency of the energy-producing microcells called mitochondria, which are present in the brain in the highest concentrations (The Charlie Foundation, n.d.).

Making the metabolic shift, i.e., burning fat for energy, is common to both intermittent fasting and the ketogenic diet. Therefore, one can say that intermittent keto will also help an average adult boost brain health within two to three weeks of following the regimen.

What if I were to tell you that even as we speak, each cell in your brain might be busy self-eating? Sounds ugly and scary, but it's the truth!

Autophagy, a Greek word that directly translates as "self-devouring," is a perfectly normal and quite essential evolutionary mechanism in our body. Dr. Priya Khorana, with a Ph.D. in Nutrition Education from Columbia University, explains, "Autophagy is the body's way of cleaning out damaged cells, to regenerate newer, healthier cells. Studies suggest that starvation-induced autophagy has neuroprotective functions" (Lindberg, 2018, para. 1-4).

Dr. Luiza Petre, a cardiologist, adds the following:

> When the body is low on sugar through fasting or ketosis, it brings the positive stress that wakes up the survival repairing mode; removing from the cells toxic proteins that are attributed to neurodegenerative diseases such as Parkinson's and Alzheimer's
>
> (Lindberg, 2018, para. 1-4).

Another interesting study revealed that the main benefit of the low-carb IF diet, outside of weight loss, is for cognitive health. Dr. Richard Isaacson, Director of the Alzheimer's Prevention Clinic at Weill Cornell Medicine and NewYork-Presbyterian Hospital in New York City said that following the low-carb, time-restricted intermittent fasting calmed down insulin pathways, letting the brain benefit from the burning of ketones as fuel. He said, "It offers great benefits for people with Alzheimer's disease." Dr. Isaacson also revealed that he personally follows the 8-hour feeding and 16-hour fasting method for four to five days a week. He strongly recommended this strategy for limiting fat accumulation around the waist: "A bigger belly might mean a smaller memory center in the brain," Dr. Isaacson explained (Migala, 2019).

Boosting Your Metabolism

Young adults in the house need to listen to this. Intermittent keto has extremely beneficial effects on the growth hormones in your body. While following intermittent keto, you may find your growth hormones increased five-fold. That sounds like really splendid news for your fat loss and muscle gain goals. While indicating a significant loss of harmful belly fat, studies have shown that intermittent keto causes less muscle loss.

Aside from that, IF + keto increases the release of the fat-burning hormone norepinephrine (noradrenaline). Due to the positive changes in hormones, short-term IF + keto may increase your metabolic rate by 3.6-14%. Intermittent keto can change the function of genes related to longevity and improve protection against disease (Gunnars, 2020).

However, like a statutory warning, I repeat: Pregnant or breastfeeding women and those with a history of eating disorders should avoid intermittent keto.

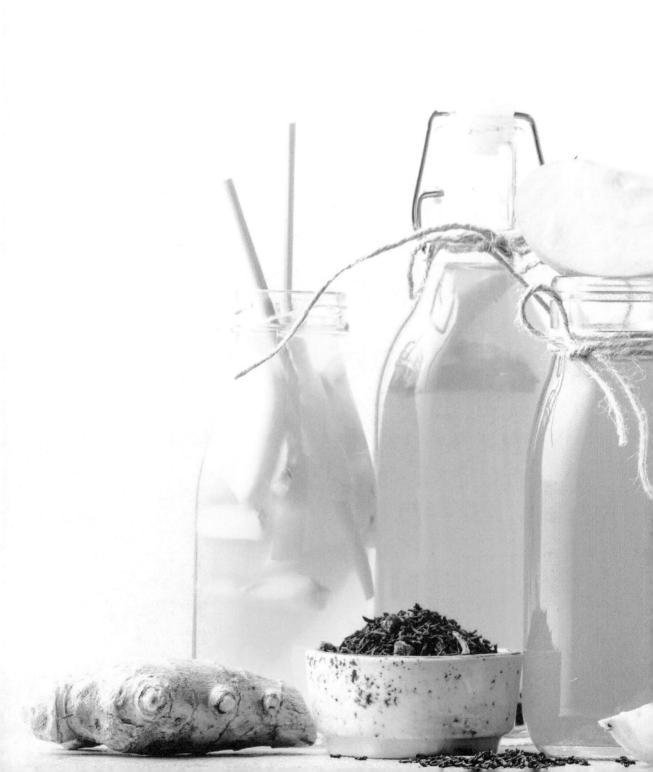

Chapter 6:
The Way to Good Gut Health—Righty-O!

You know the gastro-intestinal tract in your body by its nickname: gut. The gut and the

You've got some guts to ignore your gut health!

stomach together make your digestive system. Heartburn, constipation, bloating, and gas are all problems in your digestive system that show the overall health of your body. You cannot possibly ignore these early signs and risk developing diseases.

Johns Hopkins gastroenterologist Gerard Mullin, M.D. says, "When gut health is good, you are less likely to experience damaging inflammation and lapses in immunity." Shifts in stomach acid, gut immunity, and gastrointestinal flora—the complex ecosystem of bacteria in your intestine—are the drivers of gut health change

(Johns Hopkins Medicine, n.d.).

What to Eat for Better Gut Health While on Keto

Gut microbial communities, also known as gut microbiota and microbiome, may sound like inconspicuous parts of our digestive system, but it is actually just the opposite. They are more important than you think. Gut microbiota are the ones who have been working at the grassroots level, so to speak. They produce essential vitamins and keep you protected from many diseases.

While following intermittent keto, you need to factor in the quality of the macros in the foods you are eating. That will ensure you are not creating an imbalance in the digestive ecosystem and unknowingly destroying the good bacteria in your gut. The good news is that now there's scientific evidence that the ketogenic diet has positive effects on the health of the gut microbiota.

Observations say that diets with high-fat content, quality polyunsaturated fats, and plant-derived proteins help maintain normal gut function. Aside from being beneficial for your gut microbiomes, plant-derived proteins such as mung bean protein are good for your metabolism. Intestinal bifidobacteria and lactic acid bacteria increase when you consume a fermented prebiotic. It also acts as an energy source for colonocytes. Probiotics are living bacteria and yeasts, usually added to yogurts and used for preparing specialty food items. Adding adequate amounts of probiotics to your diet is a scientifically approved method of improving gut health.

Recently, Parmesan, an Italian dry and hard cheese, was discovered to be a great way of introducing friendly bacteria into your gut. Thus, eating even a small piece of high-fat fermented food like Parmesan cheese every day will support the colonization of the microbiota living in your gut and improve your general health, too. On the other hand, however, you must avoid using artificial sweeteners to replace natural sugars in your ketogenic diet. Several pieces of evidence have shown that artificial sweeteners affect gut microbiota negatively (Paoli et al., 2019).

Including Healthy Gut Support

Well, we know that we all have unique gut environments with different microbiota thriving there. Hence, the way each individual body will respond to intermittent keto will be very different. However, there are a couple of ways to ensure you are maintaining good gut health, and at the same time, they may also help reduce digestion-related side effects when you kick-start your keto.

Apple Cider Vinegar (ACV)

I wonder if Isaac Newton knew that the apple had more to give him than just the idea of gravity when it dropped on his head. Jokes aside, you can make the elixir of life out of apples. I call apple cider vinegar "the elixir of life" because it indeed acts as a magic potion and helps extend your life by improving your health.

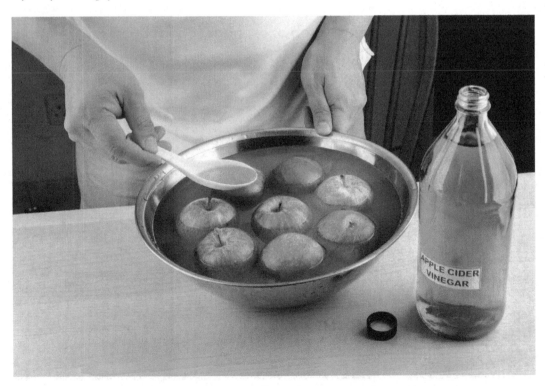

Apple cider vinegar is very well recognized for its multiple benefits and is prescribed for many health conditions. It is made by fermenting apple juice until it has turned into a hard cider. The natural sugars in the fruit get fermented into alcohol. Bacteria further ferment it and turn it into acetic acid.

A study published in *Bioscience, Biotechnology, and Biochemistry* stated that a daily dose of one tablespoon of ACV diluted in two cups of water over 12 weeks helped obese participants with body fat, weight, and waist size reduction. The acetic acid in apple cider vinegar reduces blood sugar and insulin and increases satiety. Studies have also shown that ACV boosts weight loss by increasing energy expenditure and fat burning, reducing fat storage, and slowing down the process by which the stomach empties (Rose, 2018).

Low-Carb Probiotics

Ingesting natural low-carb probiotics adds good bacteria into your digestive system that fight and reduce the bad bacteria, if any, and restore the balance in your gut microbiota.

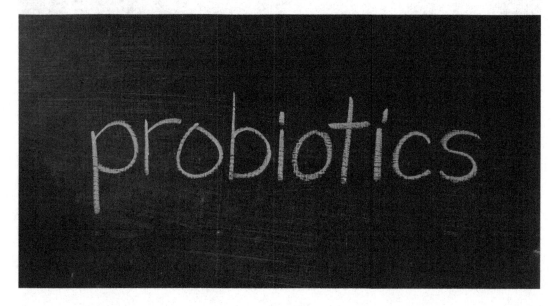

Here are some low-carb probiotics that you can include in your keto meal plan (DoctorNDTV, 2019):

1. Yogurt (Unsweetened)

A great low-carb source for good fat and protein that you can easily include in your keto meal plan. One cup of yogurt after lunch or dinner helps digestion.

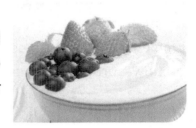

2. Sauerkraut

Made from fermented cabbage, it is a great low-carb food that is rich in fiber. Sauerkraut supplies the enzymes needed for the quick absorption of nutrients.

3. Kombucha

It is made by fermenting sweetened green or black tea with yeast. It becomes fizzy by natural fermentation methods. Even though it is sweet and fizzy, it is still a low-carb drink good for the liver and gut. You can include it in your intermittent keto diet, but keep in mind that it contains sugar, so you must count your macros accordingly.

4. Kimchi

Another popular probiotic food is kimchi made with fermented vegetables like cabbage and garlic, salt, spices, chili peppers, and vinegar. Kimchi not only helps improve digestion but can also prevent yeast infections.

5. Traditional Pickles

Made by fermenting cucumbers, the traditional pickle is fat-free and low in calories. You can enjoy pickled cucumbers while following a keto diet without a worry! The traditional pickle is a healthy probiotic that helps promote the growth of healthy bacteria in the gut.

6. Cheese

Particular types of cheese contain probiotics, like raw cheese (made from unpasteurized milk from cows, sheep, or goats) and aged cheese (such as blue cheese, Feta, cheddar, Gouda, provolone, mozzarella, and Emmental). All the cheeses have varying percentages of macros, but most are low-carb alternatives (KetoVale, 2019).

I've got a gut feeling you'll be saying" Yeeto!" for good gut health right now.

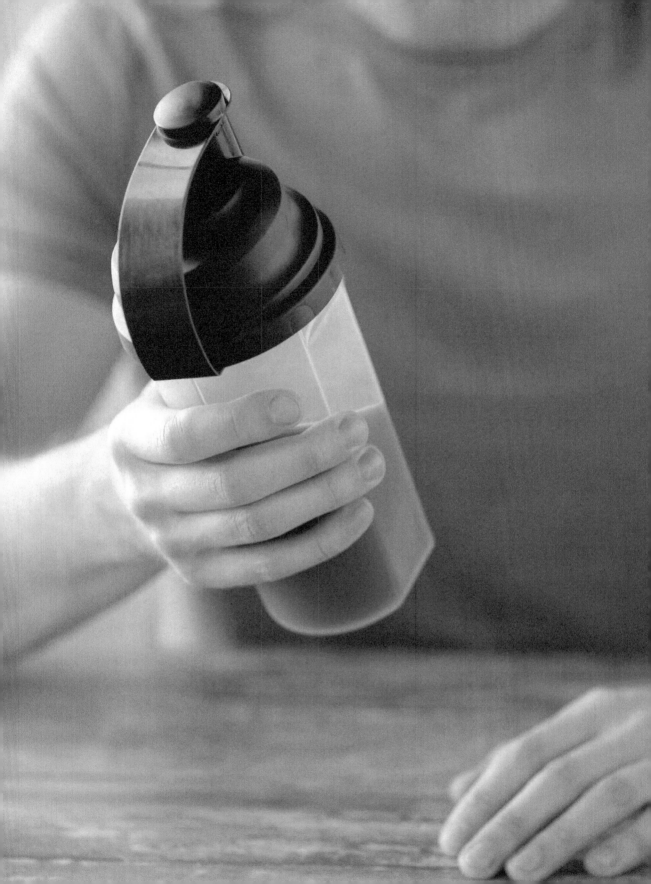

Chapter 7:

The Right Supplement Mix-O

Although even a kid at school will tell you what their mom said: you have to eat your greens. You

Are supplements beneficial for your health? Undoubtedly.

have to maintain a balanced diet to get the best nutrition. Yes, even while following keto, your health is a priority besides losing weight and burning fat.

It is an open secret that in our busy daily lives, we often overlook the health quotient of our plate. You may be counting your macros and cooking healthy meals most of the time, but on many occasions, you also appease your hunger by going with a quick mug of black coffee and maybe a handful of nuts and berries. In the long run, that will simply not do any good for your health, will it? You are maintaining ketosis and hitting the bull's-eye of staying within the daily macro budget, but unknowingly, you are going head-on toward nutrient deficiency.

The sudden metabolic switching from glucose to fats in the ketosis process also stuns your body temporarily. Like a deer blinded by the headlights, your body goes into panic mode until it can see what you are up to as a positive change. Meanwhile, you will have to bear with the side effects or try to find a way around them.

Now, you have to stay calm and stop worrying about every single thing. There are a bunch of superheroes waiting to jump into action. They are known as keto supplements. They can be the guardians of your overall health. Some supplements are especially created to minimize symptoms and side effects for keto dieters.

Just as there are different leagues of superheroes you follow avidly on screen, you will be amazed to see how many types of supplements are available out there. It's mind-boggling—so to save you from the frustration of research, experimentation, and the guessing game about which is the best one on the shelf, I will recommend a particular brand that I have come to trust over time.

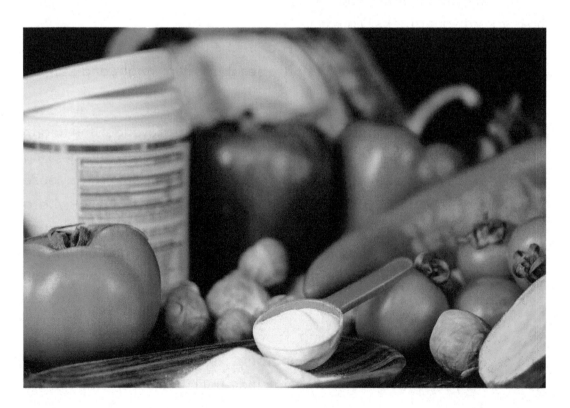

Dr. David Perlmutter, M.D., has formulated the Garden of Life Keto line of products. Their supplements are all compliant with the keto guidelines and are easy to use, delicious, and provide just the right mix of nutrients! If you know that your diet lacks a particular nutrient, visit their website and take your pick from the wide range of keto products without any worries or doubts. Their products are all clean and fully transparent, "Keto Certified," "Non-GMO Project Verified," and grass-fed (Keto Products | Garden of Life, n.d.).

When you are spoiled for choice, you tend to feel lost or waste time with indecisiveness. Let me simplify things for you. Here are some nutritional supplements that you might want to consider:

Electrolytes

During ketosis, there is an imbalance of fluids due to excessive water loss from the body. The first sign you are dehydrated is when you feel extremely thirsty from time to time. Electrolytes such as the mineral magnesium are essential for restoring the balance of fluids, smooth metabolism, maintenance of bone health, and more. Since the keto diet cuts out beans, whole grains, and some fruits, which are sources of magnesium, your body may become deficient in this important mineral.

Other electrolytes that your body needs are chloride, potassium, phosphorus, and sodium. Supplements can pump them back into your system.

Medium-Chain Triglyceride (MCT) Oil

This oil is not found in many foods except for coconut oil. Being a type of fatty acid, it is metabolized for energy. MCT oil is, therefore, regarded as an excellent aid for ketosis. Taking supplements that contain MCT oil while on keto can speed up your fat loss.

Fiber

Fiber is well-hidden in plant-based carb sources, hence, you may not be getting enough of it when you are on a strict keto diet. Even though many recommended keto-friendly foods like avocado, nuts, and seeds contain fiber, a protein-heavy diet can outweigh the fiber intake you'll need. Getting enough fiber from your foods is essential for maintaining a healthy digestive system. Keto-friendly supplements that have a fiber-rich formula will alleviate constipation, indigestion, and help clear your bowels.

L-Theanine

This amino acid reduces anxiety, keeps away depression, improves your sleep cycle, and enhances mental clarity. However, it is only available in negligible quantities in a few types of green and black teas. Some who start the keto diet begin to experience mental fog, which can affect concentration. Taking L-theanine food supplements could do wonders at chasing away the side effects and improving mental cognition.

So even if you fear that your daily keto diet is not up to your desired nutritional mark, you can visit the Garden of Life's online range of products or pick some up off the shelf of local health food stores or retail stores such as Walmart.

The Garden of Life Grass-Fed Butter Powder is one of the keto supplements you can begin with which I believe checks all the boxes as the best supplement mix.

Why Grass-Fed Butter Is Better

You might think that the story of your favorite butter started in the udder of the cow. That's only partially true. The butter you eat comes from the milk that the cow gave, but the nutrition in the milk comes from what the cow eats.

Milk is highly nutritious, as it contains various macro and micro components beneficial to human health, but apparently, the nutrition levels are influenced by the cow's diet. If you were to check, you would realize that most dairy cows are fed corn or grains. Research suggests that pasture feeding significantly improves the nutritional profile of bovine milk, so that is why the quality of the "grass-fed" milk resonates with consumers who desire healthy, organic dairy products (Alothman et al., 2019).

It was observed that grass-fed milk has 26% more omega-3 polyunsaturated fatty acids that have anti-inflammatory properties. Another analysis reported that grass-fed dairy has 500% more conjugated linoleic acid (CLA) than the regular dairy we usually consume. Thus, butter made from grass-fed milk not only has a healthier fat profile but is also believed to be loaded with vitamin K2, which plays an important role in bone and heart health. Grass-fed butter is a rich source of vitamin A and beta-carotene. While vitamin A helps increase immunity, beta-carotene is a potent antioxidant that can reduce the risk of several chronic diseases (Meixner, 2019).

Now that you have realized the nutritional value of replacing your regular butter with grass-fed butter, I'm sure you will be seeking it out. At the same time, it would be good to remind yourself that it is still butter with the artery-clogging cholesterols we fear.

Thus comes into play the importance of using the Garden of Life Grass Fed Butter Powder. It will not only supply vitamins, minerals, medium-chain triglyceride (MCT) oil, and omega-3 fatty acids but is also a source of 1.5 billion CFU probiotics. It does not contain any antibiotics.

Aside from being a health supplement, it also tastes delicious. It's perfect for youth who are perpetually on the go or busier than bees and is easy to mix into your daily cup of tea, coffee, or your keto milkshakes and smoothies.

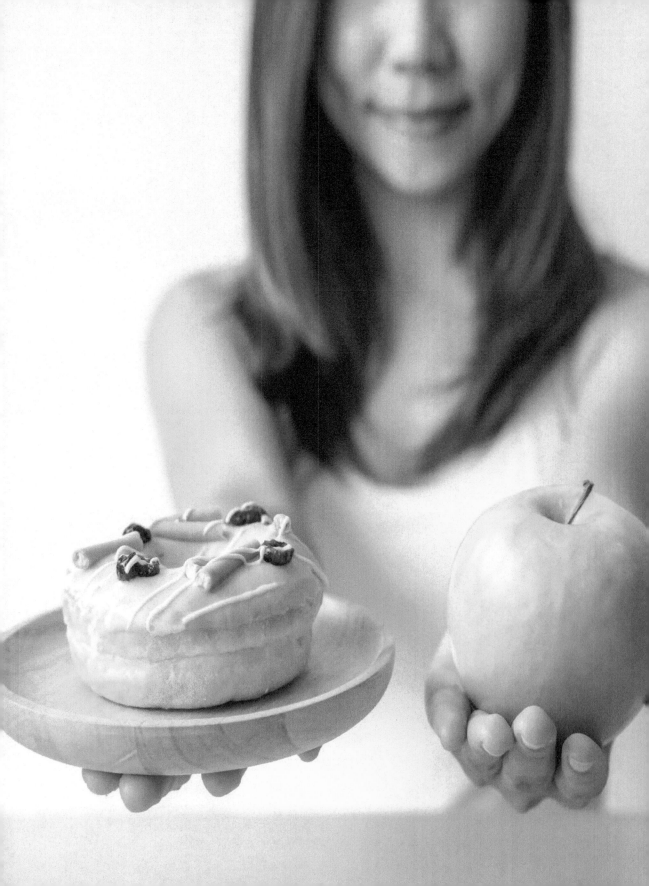

Chapter 8:
Strategize Your Weight Loss—Cheat-O!

This is one of those rare occasions when you will be schooled in cheating. Cheating will be strategized, discussed, and debated. You are going to be told how cheating is a legitimate move. Can life get shadier than this? This is the thug life!

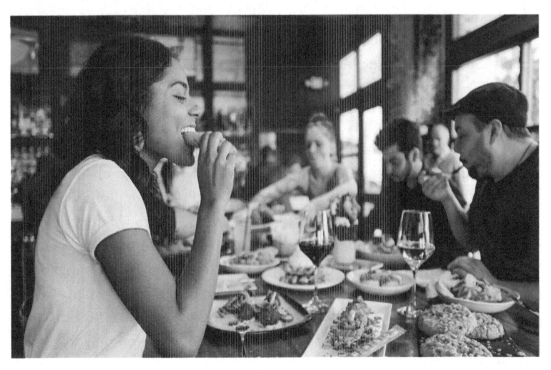

The initial phase of adjusting to keto is undeniably tough for many, and it is natural to feel tempted to break the rule once in a while. Sometimes, you may even feel like quitting on your fat-burning mission completely: The struggle is real!

To save yourself from falling off the weight-loss wagon, you try to devise plans. You sneak a sweet snack. Once in a while, you take a slice of the pizza that the others are enjoying, and then, you burn with guilt. Instead of focusing on burning that fat, you are wallowing in self-pity. I feel you, but going down that road is not going to help at all.

So let's bring a method to the madness with another tried-and-tested formula that will help you cheat yourself into sticking with the diet, free you of guilt, let you live your life with keto, and not struggle to exist!

The simplest way to stay on top of your keto game is to learn when and how to cheat in a planned manner. Once you have started experiencing the tremendous weight loss and health benefits of the ketogenic diet, I can imagine you will be ready to do anything to get to your weight loss goals. So let us strategize how best to cheat-o!

Weekly Cheat Meal vs. Cheat All Day

The idea of cheat meals or the cheat day was created after the psychology of a dieter was better understood. Ever since childhood, we have all been conditioned to run for the reward. All Olympians work hard and bear through rigorous training until the leap year to win that coveted gold medal. The difference here is that you are competing with your own willpower. One trick is to develop a reward system for motivation to continue and stick to the strict keto diet. Give yourself something to look forward to. Promise yourself a treat as soon as you have hit a particular mark with your weight loss. However, it is crucial that you only treat—not overeat.

There are two popular reward systems: the cheat meal or the cheat day. Either you promise yourself one cheat meal consisting of any food you really want to eat, or you could decide on one cheat day when you go off keto and eat whatever you like all day.

While both options sound tempting, each has its own pros and cons. It is for you to decide which reward system suits you best. What will make you happy enough to say "Yeeto!" for keto again and get back on the fat-burning train with full conviction?

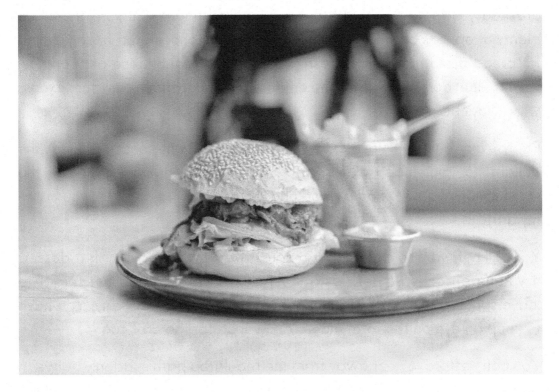

The Cheat Meal

The rule of thumb for planning your cheat meal is that you must strike off what you have been craving to eat all the while. It is most natural that something you are told NOT to eat will keep playing on your mind, so to get your mind off it, you eat it.

However, cheating does not mean knocking yourself out with junk food. That's still a NO! You know your body way better than I do, but trust me, junk food has not done any good to anyone. Despite knowing that, if you must eat that greasy burger from the local fast-food chain outlet or guzzle sodas by the case, then do it at your own risk. You would be sending all your hard work down the drain for just one moment of gratification and would then have a lot of time to regret it later.

Instead, you could plan a fun and delicious cheat meal that won't drastically affect your health or your macro budget. I'm sure there are plenty of options out there. If you choose pizza, choose the freshly baked flatbread pizza made with fresh produce and real cheese as toppings. Take a slice; don't wolf down the entire pan. Moderation is a virtue; excess will always be a vice.

Enjoy every bite, the flavors, and the taste. Let your senses register the delight to remember it for later. Everything that will trigger the satisfaction of having had a good cheat meal—your reward. Do you catch my drift?

You will not want to desert your macros even while enjoying that dessert if you have accepted keto as a lifestyle change. Also, do not forget to leave space for another meal or some snacks later in the day. You have to keep an eye on the total macro allowance for the day, too.

You can't afford to veer away from the regulated path suddenly between your keto mission. That doesn't mean I'm asking you to calculate and set a strict calorie budget for the cheat meal, too. It should indeed take the pressure off you, but you cannot entirely forsake eating responsibly. Have fun but don't overdo it is all that I meant to say. Your cheat meal should be a strategic move and not a detrimental misstep.

If you are following intermittent keto, it could work in your favor here. You could time the cheat meal within your eating cycle. That way, your cheat meal will not be doing too much harm. You could eat guilt-free while you are still on your fat-burning mission.

There's also the theory that a cheat meal can be a great tool to pull yourself out when you have hit a plateau with your weight loss. When on keto, your body is burning fat for energy, but there comes a point when it starts protecting its fat reserves, and your progress stalls. In such situations, you are advised to lessen your calorie intake to continue losing weight. The drastic drop in calorie intake is also unhealthy. This is where a cheat meal will be appropriate. If you eat a high-calorie cheat meal that supplies enough calories from the good macros, you will be preventing your metabolism from slowing down.

Plus, someone said something ages ago about not being able to have the cake and eat it, too!

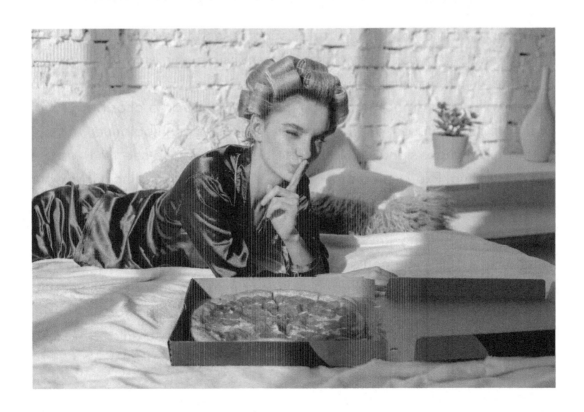

The Cheat Days

Give yourself one whole day to break free from the keto restrictions. I hope that did not sound like a license to binge eat for an entire day. Eat as many meals as you wish, and eat whatever you like, but be kind to yourself. Avoid those unhealthy junk foods and sugary drinks. There's always a natural, healthier source that will satiate your cravings.

The purpose of the cheat day is to simply take a day off to recharge your batteries and resume your mission with renewed energy—quite literally. What you are essentially doing on a cheat day is that you are supplying your body with its old source of energy: carbs. You are shaking your metabolism up again and thus putting it back to work. A cheat day can thereby do wonders not only for your psychology but also for the physical progress of your fat-burning mission. The massive advantage of planning a cheat day is that it can help you override a weight-loss plateau.

However, as I told you before, ketosis increases the synthesis of leptin—the hormone in your body that is responsible for suppressing your appetite. Simultaneously, your body is also running low on ghrelin, which prevents the urge to eat more. It is most likely that on a cheat day, your body will get confused, as the hormones will be in an imbalance. Without the natural hunger signals, you have to be more alert to see that you are not overeating. Exercise control over the portions and helpings of all your meals throughout the cheat day.

If you are practicing intermittent keto, you can enjoy your cheat day without any guilt. You could choose to follow the alternate-day fasting method and see that your cheat day coincides with your eat day. Keep to clean eating and stay within the daily calorie budget. Thus, you would still be on your weight-loss mission even as you eat what you enjoy the most. It wouldn't feel like you are cheating anymore!

Making Cheat-O a Winning Strategy

Whether it is the cheat meal or the cheat day, it will work to your advantage only if you follow certain disciplines. Here are some tips for doing it right:

➢ Decide if it's going to be a cheat meal or a cheat day and stick with it.

➢ See that it doesn't suddenly go from one cheat meal to an entire cheat day or stretch into a cheat week that turns into a cheat month all on a whim.

➢ Gearing up for a cheat day or a cheat meal does not mean starving yourself for it. Do not pounce on a large meal with an empty stomach.

➢ Cheat meals and cheat days should be an indulgence. Do not send yourself on a guilt trip after that. Refocus and get back to work with intermittent keto.

➢ Strategy means a planned approach. Plan your cheat meal and plan every meal on your cheat day, so you can derive the maximum benefit from it. Thus, the results will also not be random or unexpected.

➢ Last but not least, listen to your body as it gives you signs. It tells you if a cheat meal is working in your favor or not. You can change your strategy accordingly if you have taken note of the details.

There is no one-size-fits-all kind of solution available here. One cannot be deemed a better winning strategy than another. Anything that works for me may not work for my own sibling, so recommending the cheat day over the cheat meal or vice versa would be impractical and downright wrong. You must keep a keen eye on how your body responds to the slightest change in your diet plan.

The cheat meal versus the cheat day cannot be debated. Both are known to have been effective strategies for innumerable people. There is, however, a proven scientific explanation as to why cheat days work.

In 1978, Brickman and others conducted research to arrive at the Set Point Theory of Subjective Well-Being, which suggests that every individual has a default level of happiness that we automatically drop back to after a prolonged period. When we start, we may feel happy with the fabulous results that the ketogenic diet gives us. Progressively, however, the initial excitement of switching to the new lifestyle, learning new recipes, and seeing the numbers on the scale move will die down, and we will begin to feel less happy with everything. We may feel a tad bored with the routine, too. This stage is also known as hedonic adaptation ("Hedonic treadmill," 2019).

The *Journal of Consumer Psychology*, flagged by *BPS Research Digest*, published reports that cheat days act as planned hedonic deviations which boost your drive to continue. It was also observed that those given the option to splurge a bit on cheat days showed more self-control while dieting. Also, they came up with more strategies to overcome temptations even though they were on a stricter diet plan (Khazan, 2016).

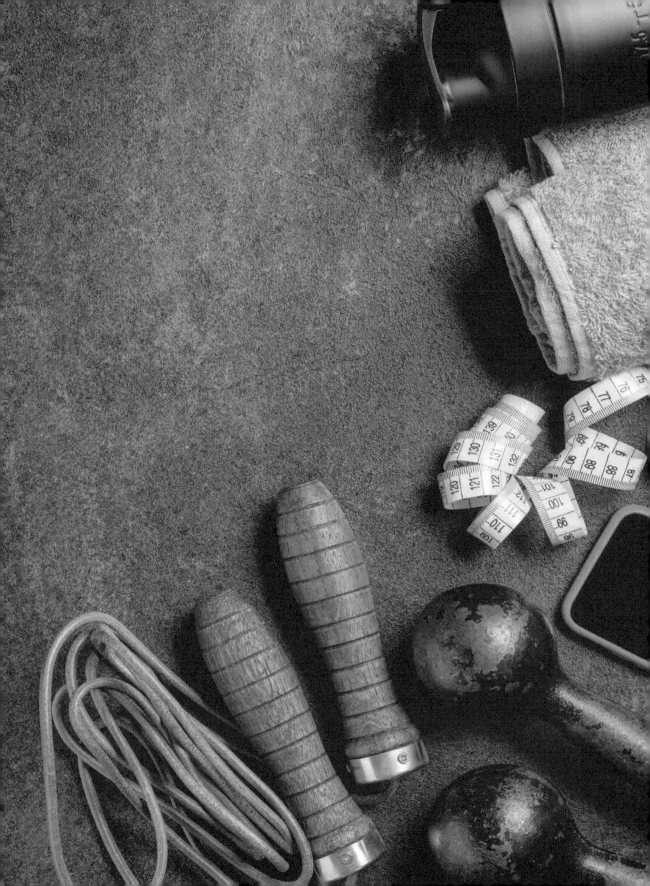

Chapter 9:

Basic, Low-Impact Exercises to Get Fit-O

Fat shaming is a big no-no, but fat burning is a big YES, right? Then, why don't we do the routine? Fist bump? Dance a jig? Well, you could do that—but before that, yell "Yeeto for keto!" then, take some steps to get "Fit-O" on your journey!

While ketosis is busy on the inside, why don't we get busy on the outside? While the excess fat is melting away, you are discovering a new you. A little light exercise just might add that extra touch and bring forth a fitter-looking you. Some basic, low-impact exercises also help you with other areas such as mental health—acting as de-stressors, improving your sleep patterns, reducing anxiety, and keeping away depression.

Do not start with an intensive routine from the get-go. Simply sitting less and moving more throughout your day is enough to show you some benefits in the initial days. "Something is always better than nothing" should be your motto when you begin developing your daily exercise routine, and then, let it gradually grow on you! You will enjoy it more when you experience the fantastic changes that even a little low-impact exercise can bring to your body and mind. Then, you will automatically want to do more in your exercise routine. Stay active for most days and give yourself a rest day.

For substantial health benefits, though, government guidelines in the U.S., U.K., and other countries recommend that you engage in moderate-intensity activity for at least 150 minutes per week. That's 30 minutes a day for five days each week. You could break it down into 10-minute sessions if that's easier (Robinson, 2019).

Then, depending on how much your body will permit you to do, you could consider intensifying your exercise regimen. Combine three or more types of exercises of your choice to develop a well-rounded daily workout routine. Aerobics, brisk walking, dancing, or cycling combined with strength training will do the trick. You could even throw in some yoga or Pilates to improve your flexibility. Each exercise session should comprise a decided number of sets of reps.

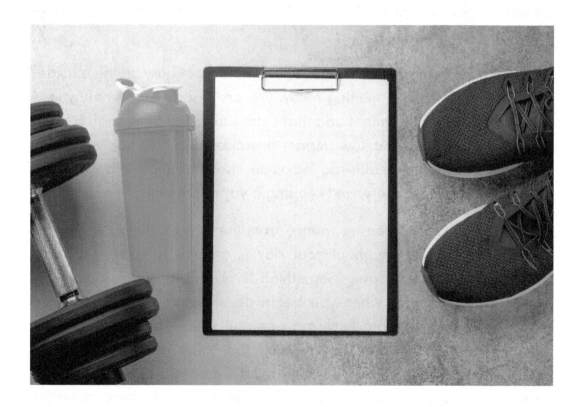

Sets and Reps

These are commonly used terms in the context of exercising. When you repeat a particular exercise, it is referred to as a "rep." When you repeat the same exercise a specific number of times, you have performed one "set" of many reps. You take a break of at least 30 seconds between multiple sets.

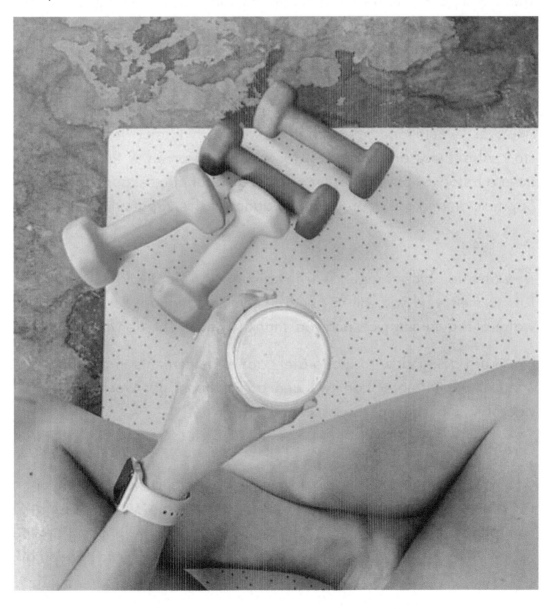

Basic Moderate-Intensity Exercises

Your motto at this point should be to remember that everything you do needs to be for YOU. This should set the tone to motivate you into moving, and you could remember it for your dear friend, Keto. Many low-intensity exercises can launch you into ketosis.

The low-impact cardio exercises can get your heart pumping, and at the same time, they will go easy on your joints. You don't need sophisticated equipment to start an exercise routine, and you could very well do it from the comfort of your home.

You can easily find a good tutorial of every exercise on YouTube. However, I would recommend that you work with a fitness instructor at the start. Also, these are not meant for pregnant women or those who may have a history of physical trauma. You could, of course, consult a doctor or physician and get appropriate guidance in this direction.

Aerobics

Try water aerobics or regular—both can be very effective at getting those fats to melt, and you will not end up feeling fatigued. Keep sipping on water at regular intervals and you, thankfully, won't be dehydrated either.

If you are doing slow to moderately active movements in aerobics, you need to put in more than two and a half hours per week, but if it is vigorous, 75 minutes per week should do.

Cycling

Cycling is also quite beneficial for your heart. Use a stationary cycle or go for a ride down the street: The effect will be the same. Start at a comfortable pace; as you get comfortable with your weight and cycling becomes a routine, your pace will gradually improve. The faster you go, the better results you will see. Let the progress be smooth, though. Do not try to forcibly accelerate if your body does not feel like it is ready for it.

Floor Exercises

If you are the type who gets bored doing the same exercise for a long time, then basic floor exercises can be your best bet. Create small sessions of 10–15 minutes of a fixed number of sets and reps.

Pick a few floor exercises like crunches, jumping jacks, pushups, squats, etc. Do one exercise for just a minute and immediately follow it up with a minute of the next exercise without a break. After completing a circuit of six exercises, take a break for a minute, and repeat it all over again one more time. Your 15-minute regimen of low-impact cardio is done.

Pilates

This is a highly recommended exercise for strengthening your core and even improving your flexibility without straining your joints. It's ideal for those who have desk jobs as it is a great way to correct your posture.

Swimming

If you ask me, there is no better cardio than a few laps in the swimming pool. The results also begin to show immediately. Make it part of a regular routine and you can be sure you are fit inside and out. It's a one-stop shop of sorts. Swimming improves flexibility, strengthens muscles and joints, tones your entire body, and keeps your mind happy and your heart healthy.

Tai Chi

A gentle form of exercise, Tai Chi is a great way of improving your physical and mental health. It will appear more like a dance form with its fluid hand movements and graceful poses. Tai Chi improves your sense of balance; it is sure to have an absolutely calming effect on you. As a bonus, Tai Chi could also help improve sleep cycles and alleviate depression and anxiety.

Walking

Walking is arguably the most underestimated form of cardio. Since it is the most basic ability given to man, we take it for granted and do not engage in enough of it. Walking after meals should be made mandatory for good health.

If you are considering walking as an exercise with or without a treadmill, increase your pace gradually. Do not try to walk at top speed in the first weeks; also, do not walk for too long. Short sessions are perfectly fine. You can increase intensity after a few weeks when you are really comfortable. Start walking on an incline, increase the pace, and try to walk for a longer time.

You could also consider running if you feel fit enough for it. However, remember running on an incline will put pressure on your joints, so consider it carefully before you include it in your daily exercise routine.

Yoga

Yoga is arguably the most misunderstood form of cardio. Depending on the yoga pose and the number of times you repeat it, yoga can give varied and impressive results. The Surya Namaskar is the most popular and recommended set of yoga exercises. It is not only gentle on the joints but also powerful and rejuvenating.

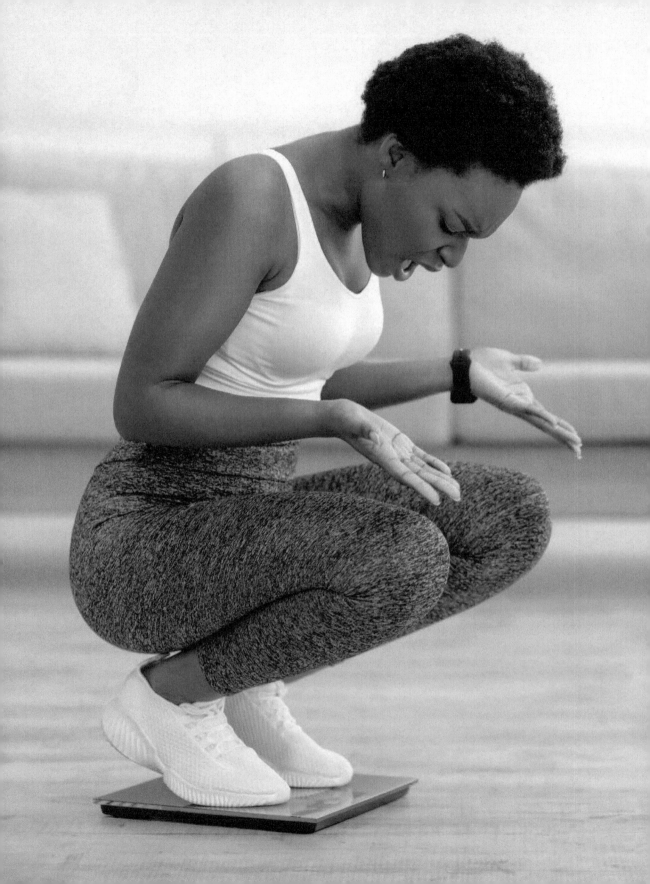

Chapter 10:

Yeeto Hacks—What to Do
If You Plateau

A weight-loss plateau is like inadvertently hitting the pause button on your weight-loss process. You cannot understand why, but the weight loss you were seeing until recently has come to a halt. Even if you're still doing everything precisely as per the weight-loss regimen, nothing seems to be working anymore. You may feel perturbed, but let's look at it from another perspective.

Imagine, you are out on a road trip, driving along and enjoying the changing scenery. Would you have liked it if it was smooth roads throughout? The thrill is in the twists and turns as well as the ups and downs. The varying topography makes the journey interesting, doesn't it?

You should expect something similar out of your keto journey, too. It's going to be a learning curve sometimes, and you just might have to be on the alert and negotiate an unexpected pothole. However, let's curb the philosophical and talk about a practical problem that is a dreaded possibility in your keto journey.

The plateau. What must you do if you have reached it? I say that you should first find out why you have hit the plateau, and then, figuring out how to get out of there will be way simpler.

What Might Have Caused the Plateau?

Everything is perfectly fine in your keto life until you see that your weight loss has stalled. Hitting a plateau is quite a common phenomenon, but knowing that you aren't alone isn't much of a consolation.

You can begin analyzing your situation by first confirming whether you have really hit a plateau. Sometimes, it may only *seem* like a plateau. If you see even the most minimal weight loss daily, you haven't arrived at a plateau yet. Your metabolism slows down after losing considerable weight through long-term food restriction. Subsequently, your body goes into the automatic mode of protecting its fat reserves. As a consequence, less fat or calories are being burned daily.

You could switch from watching your weight daily to observing a pattern in weight loss at the end of every week. Do not jump to the conclusion that you have indeed hit a plateau until it has been over three months of having no marked weight loss—despite having continued with the keto diet.

Various factors influence weight loss, beginning with the weighing scale you use for your exercise regimen, medical history, or even your sleep cycles.

Sometimes, it may so happen that you have metabolic problems, high stress levels, or sleep and hunger issues that may interfere with your weight loss. In such situations, you must adapt to a new weight-loss strategy or change it completely.

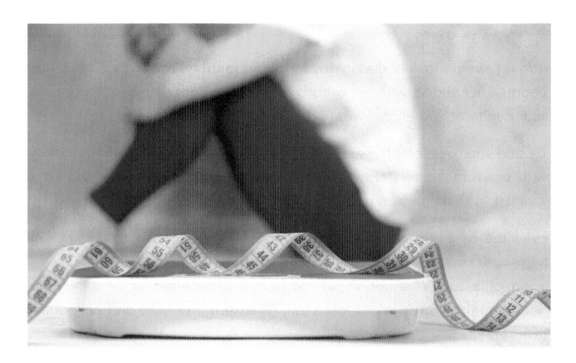

Yeeto Hacks

Here are some science-backed hacks that might help you drive out of a plateau at top speed:

1. Hunt for Hidden Carbs

If you are not calculating your macros regularly, carbs can quietly slip into your diet and hide away from your sight. Out with the stowaways! You may find them hidden in foods such as sausages, deli meats, salad dressings, gravies and sauces, processed and packaged goods, or even products that are touted as keto-friendly. You need to read the labels carefully and study the macro specifications.

Have you, by any chance, included high-carb vegetables like carrots, squash, and red onions on your menu? Recheck that you have crossed off high-carb fruits from your grocery list and totally shed the habit of drinking fruit juices. How often do you eat berries? Scale down or cut them out from your diet completely to start seeing results from keto once again.

2. Skip the Sweet Treats

Adding sweets to your diet in any form or quantity is not a good idea. Just because it's made with a no-carb sweetener doesn't make it good for your health or your diet. Sweets are a trigger for your cravings.

Try and skip over the offers of tempting fares like desserts and other items with a sweet base. Delay gratification as much as possible and treat yourself to them only on rare and special occasions.

Even the revolutionary idea of creating low-carb foods to mimic their high-carb versions—like muffins, cheesecakes, ice creams, breads, etc.— is an epic fail. Whether those foods are sweetened or not, they are detrimental to your weight loss plan, give zero nutrition, and only cause overeating.

3. Go Slow with Dairy and Nuts

Full-fat dairy and most nuts are suitable for inclusion in your keto diet, but too much of anything good is bad enough, isn't it? Rich cheeses or extra cream in your coffee are very easy to overdo without realizing you are doing it. However, you could completely avoid the items just as easily, so take stock and stop that right away to get out of the plateau.

You could tell yourself that you will stop at just one nut but then end up gobbling a few of that tasty, salty goodness. Reduce or remove dairy and nuts from your daily intake, and you just might get a historic breakthrough.

4. Curb That Urge for Snacking

Is there a quick snack on your mind? Curb that urge. It is the first sign that your daily meals are not giving you sufficient amounts of protein, or the fats in your meals are not supplying enough energy.

Your low-carb meals plan should be good enough to keep you from feeling hungry for four to five hours straight. If that's not happening, try to add macros to your meals while staying within your daily allowance.

However, snacking once in a while is still a bad idea, as it can grow into a habit and hamper your weight loss. Remember: Every carb and calorie adds to the total—even if it is a low-carb bite or a keto-friendly snack.

5. Pack in Precise Protein

Too much protein on your plate can add more calories than you need to your diet, and too little will leave you feeling hungry which is responsible for triggering the urge for snacking, and then you find yourself overeating. Stick with the ideal keto macros formula and use the calculator to help you get back on track. It is the protein that helps you maintain your resting metabolic rate by preserving muscle mass, so it is essential to consume appropriate amounts of the macros. Be precise.

6. Don't Load Up on Fats

Fat intake should also be exactly within the prescribed keto macros budget. Remind yourself of the keto basics. Fat is the only reason why a keto diet is so satiating, but unknowingly, you could be overloading the fats on your menu. If you have hit a plateau with your weight loss, cut back on the fat intake.

If you keep feeling hungry between meals, consider making the next meal of the day heavier with fats. Ideally, add some high-quality protein to your plate, like eggs or tuna salad. You could, of course, look for a vegetarian option if you wish.

7. Impact Carbs vs. Non-impact Carbs

Impact carbs are those simple carbs that get immediately broken down into glucose which then gets stored in your liver to be used as fuel.

Whereas non-impact carbs are those complex carbs that come from fiber and sugar alcohol that pass through your body without affecting your glucose levels.

Thus, while calculating your macros, you can find out the net carbs by subtracting the grams of fiber and sugar alcohol from the total grams of carbohydrates consumed. Pay attention to what types of carbs you are consuming.

"Broccoli has just 2 grams of net carbs per ½ cup, which makes it a major superfood that should be a staple on the keto diet," says Suzanne Dixon, R.D. It's high in fiber and protein which will keep you feeling full. You can use it in just about anything: stews, soups, and keto makeovers of your favorite foods like a casserole (Baum, 2020).

8. Ration That Alcohol

Most people who follow the keto diet indulge in wines and alcoholic beverages occasionally, and that is okay. However, since alcohol gets metabolized first, consumption of high amounts will slow down the process of ketosis. Overindulgence in alcohol can not only stall but also regress your weight loss. Consuming alcohol is equivalent to guzzling unnecessarily extra, nonnutritious calories in the liquid form.

9. Don't Underestimate Stress and Sleep

It's a widespread misconception that food is the only factor influencing weight loss. Poor sleep cycles and high stress levels can cause your cortisol levels to rise and give you false hunger cues. Many times, people slip into binge eating despite all of their good intentions. Therefore, it is expected that you will see obesity and accumulating belly fat in those who are experiencing high stress levels or are sleep-deprived.

Observe your stress levels and sleep patterns to help take corrective measures. Focus on developing a good sleep routine. Start taking walks to help lower cortisol levels in the body and make you feel good. Engage in stress reduction practices such as deep breathing exercises and yoga, and revive your hobbies. I'm sure it would prove therapeutic.

10. Start Regular Exercise

Just a bit of brisk walking daily could also go a long way to improve your health and help you burn more energy.

Be sure to do your exercise before your first meal or before dinner because your insulin is low at that time. Exercise timed right can push your body to start burning through its fat stores again.

If you think you need more physical exertion to get those fats melting again, you could go for high-intensity interval training (HIIT). Resistance training such as lifting weights can get you burning more fat daily. In the meantime, you can also build some muscle and improve your resting metabolism.

11. Combine Intermittent Fasting with Keto

This one is like the trump card of all hacks! Combining keto with intermittent fasting can be a great strategic move for your weight loss.

Precisely planned nutrient-rich meals can keep you feeling full for several hours, but intermittent fasting can speed you toward ketosis. Once you are fat-adapted, your body will be ready to take on intermittent fasting, too.

Try the meal-skipping method for starters, which most find the easiest to get used to. You could also try the alternate-day IF method, where you fast one day and eat the next day the way you usually do. This could help avoid the slowing down of your metabolism. This could be the surefire solution for your weight-loss plateau.

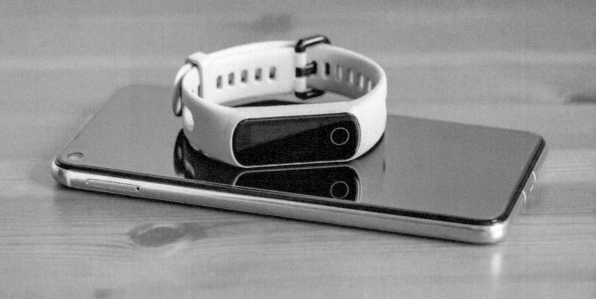

Chapter 11:
Track Your Success Daily from the Get-Go

How many times have you read a fitness article online? Don't they mostly always talk about how hard it is to get fit? Some sound as if it is a near-impossible feat to achieve. There are contradictory articles on keto, too.

Once someone realizes you are on keto, news begins to float to you via word of mouth. You may even hear your own friends tell you tales about how someone somewhere learned that the keto lifestyle is crazy and that another one threw in the proverbial towel on their weight-loss regimen. These are unnecessary distractions that can be discouraging.

Like an athlete is told to stay in their own lane, interference should not be tolerated. You must not let others affect your plan or your willingness and determination to do it. Compete with yourself. Do not make it into a race that it is definitely not!

Think less about what others are up to or how they fared with keto. Each individual has a different physiology and body tendency. Many factors affect one's success with keto, so keep a tab on what your body tells you about the keto regimen you are following. How you feel about it yourself is what really matters. Focus on your own progress and track your success.

Steps to Tracking Your Keto Success

Daily Macros Calculator

You begin by finding out your ideal daily calorie budget and recording your daily macro intake for weight loss. There are many calculators available online that can spare you the pain of doing it manually. Simply select weight loss as your keto diet goal and then provide your personal physical statistics and level of physical activity. You should have your total calorie goal and daily macro intake in grams within no time.

With keto, fat will always be the macro in the spotlight. This sets your diet apart from the low-carb lifestyle, where the macros distribution is also flexible. Remember, the winning macros formula for you is 70% fat, 25% protein, and only 5% carbs.

Here is a link to a macros calculator for you to check out:

https://ketogenic.com/calculator/

Alternatively, you could consult a dietician for it, as well.

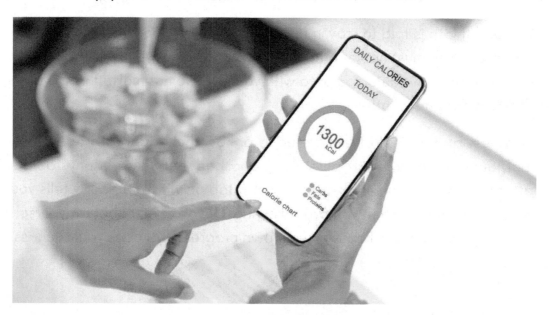

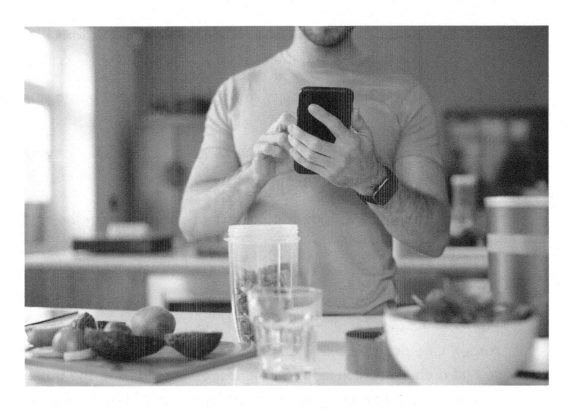

✖ myfitnesspal

Steps to Set Up MyFitnessPal

Now that you know your daily nutrition goals, you must track your progress daily. I would recommend MyFitnessPal as the best app for recording your daily calorie intake from every meal, tracking your exercise, and even maintaining a log of your physical measurements. However, you must see that your inputs are correct. You can also easily sync it with other apps for greater accuracy in inputs.

Although the free version has many features, your keto life will be much easier with the premium plan. It won't burn a hole in your pocket, so don't worry!

Here's the step-by-step method for setting yourself up for keto success with MFP (Caveman Keto, 2012):

1. Start by signing up for an account with your email address at www.myfitnesspal.com and then set up your account.

2. MyFitnessPal will then take you to settings, and you can update your personal profile.

3. From "My Home," you need to go to "Goals" and set up "Your Fitness Goals" by editing each box.

4. See that you key in your daily calorie goal acquired from the keto calculator in the box that says, "Daily Nutrition Goal." Set the "Macronutrients" as per the winning keto formula of 5% carbohydrates, 75% fat, and 20% protein.

5. Edit the "Fitness Goal" box and set the Calories Burned/Week target. One pound is 3,500 calories. I would set the weekly target to half a pound, which is 1,750 calories. You could raise the bar or lessen the target as per your personal weight-loss goal or according to what your dietician recommends.

6. Next, from "My Home," you need to go to "Check-In" and enter your "Other Measurements": neck, waist, hips, thighs, chest, and arms.

7. Then, you need to go to "Food" (the option next to "My Home"), and under "Settings" you will find a column called "Nutrients Tracked." You can maintain the order of the macros as per importance in the keto diet. Also, add fiber as the fourth macro. The last one can be any macro of your choice.

8. To enhance your MyFitnessPal user experience, you will have to do the following:

   ➤ Visit https://github.com/Surye/mfp-keto-userscript

   ➤ Download a special script that will add the **"Net Carbs"** option to your measurement statistics. To install the script, you will also have to install **Greasemonkey** (in case you use the Firefox browser) or **Tampermonkey** (if you are on Chrome).

➢ After the installation of the script is complete, you will see that you now have three additional columns:

- Net Carbs
- Carb / Fat / Protein percentages for each meal / total
- Pie chart showing percentage of calories for Carb / Fat / Protein

Track Your Meals

Under the "Food" option, you will find the "Food Diary" where you can track all your meals, including breakfast, lunch, dinner, and snacks. When you click on "Add Food," you will get the option to search their food database by name; for example, if you search for "Scrambled Eggs," you will see many options. Select one from the "Matching Foods." You get two options in the sidebar: "Add Food to Diary" and "Check Nutrition Info."

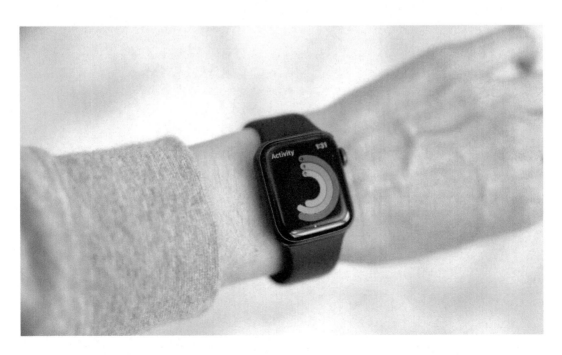

Before tracking all your meals, you must plan all the meals for the day based on the macro nutrition info. You do not want to end up with a very minimal calorie budget left on hand at the end of the day. Without a good dinner, you cannot expect to get some quality sleep. Calorie misappropriation can cause a lot of inconveniences.

This is just the start. It will take some time to get the hang of MFP and how you can use it for optimum benefit. Study the graphs and pie charts, and the more you use all the features, the more you will find it easy to fine-tune your progress.

Give us a "Yeeto!" when you begin to see the correlation between the exercises and meals you track and the fat you burn in terms of inches on your waist or the digits on your scale.

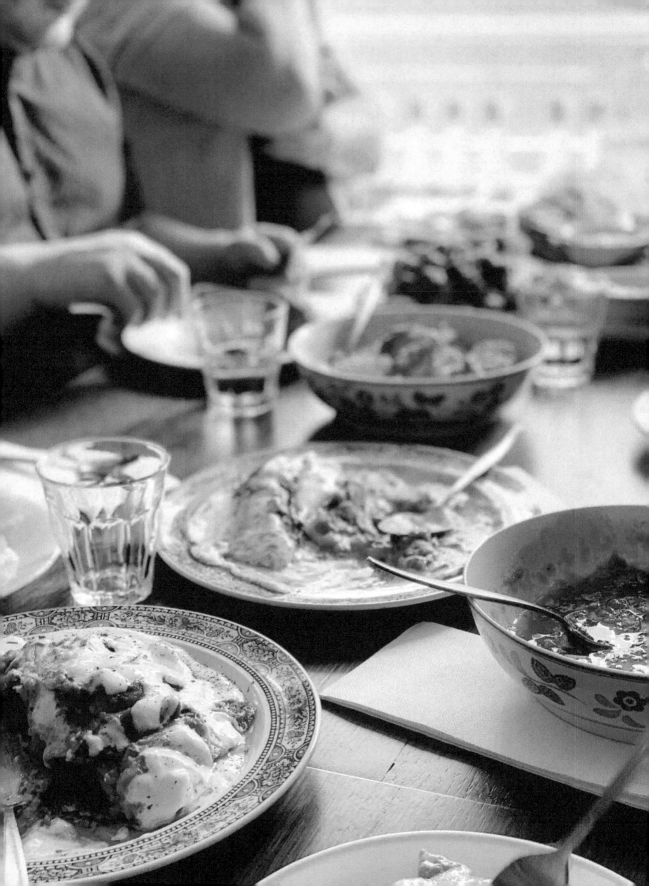

Chapter 12:

Guide to Eat-O

The ketogenic diet is known to improve your metabolism and reduce your appetite. Some homemade ketogenic diet recipes are made up of foods that will keep you feeling full for a long while. Not feeling hungry is in itself a constructive step toward faster weight loss. However, your equation with food changes entirely when you are eating out.

Temptation is indeed a vice. It can be stronger when you are hanging out in the company of friends or family. Think about it: There are restaurants, parties, and a buffet at a wedding or other ceremonies with people mindlessly loading their plates and stomachs with foods that look yummier than ever. Unfortunately, if you happen to be in the vicinity of fast food, you have to use strong determination to look away.

This pain point is common with most dieters and fitness enthusiasts. Your social life or even work life often involves eating out, and eating out ends up becoming a tiresome tug-of-war between what to eat and what not to eat.

In a recent user survey conducted by MyFitnessPal, it was observed that almost 50% of all users ate out at least once per week. While over 80% were finding it difficult to make healthy food decisions at restaurants, nearly 80% were browsing the MFP database for nutrition info before placing their order (MyFitnessPal, 2016).

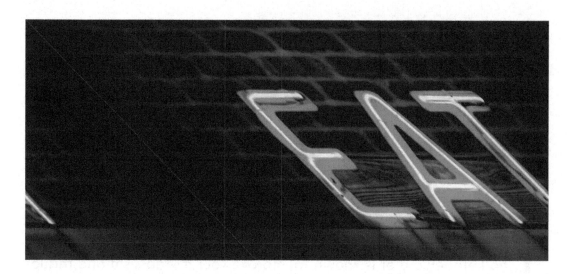

How to Eat Out

A little bit of planning can go a long way. What better guide than MyFitnessPal to show you the most keto-friendly way with your eating-out endeavor?

The best user-centric move by MFP was adding a fabulous new feature recently: "Restaurant Logging" which is available for both iOS and Android devices.

With this update, you can now quickly open the MyFitnessPal app on your smartphone from any restaurant you are eating at and add items from the menu to the log within the app. Before you place your order, you can even browse their database for the food and view the calories and macros in it. Nutrition information from menus of over 500,000 restaurants nationwide is available in their database. Despite that, if you still can't see the item from the menu in the MFP database, you can always request an addition.

You can access the map of nearby restaurant menus at a glance to select a meal option that is the best fit for your calorie and macro goals for the day (MyFitnessPal, 2016).

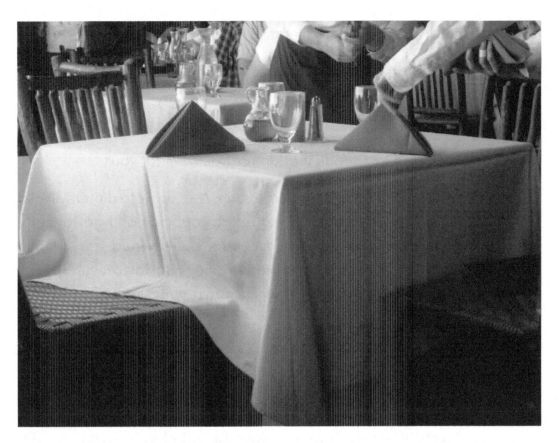

Steps to Accessing the Restaurant Logging Feature:

1. Open the MyFitnessPal app on your device.

2. Tap the blue + button at the bottom.

3. Tap on the "Food" option.

4. Look for the meal you wish to log.

5. There's a location icon to the right of the search bar. Tap on it for restaurant logging, and you're done!

Eating out without straying away from your keto diet couldn't get much easier than that!

What to Eat and What Not to Eat

If it's a last-minute decision you need to make, it feels like you really have to quickly place your order or be ready to go hungry for the rest of your road trip.

Here's a list of some fast foods that do not spell evil for you:

- Eat the patty and ditch the burger bun. A smart keto dieter will also ask for replacements of the high-carb toppings and go for keto-friendly condiments such as avocado, boiled/fried eggs, mayo, mustard, plain onion rings, salsa, lettuce, and tomatoes. Sprinkle salt and pepper to taste. Wash it down with unsweetened iced green tea.

- Order an "Unwich": Ask for the contents of a healthy chicken or tuna sandwich to be given to you wrapped in lettuce leaves.

- Request a customized keto-friendly burrito bowl without the rice and beans. What you have is a delicious salad to enjoy without any guilt. Top your bowl up with high-fat, low-carb condiments of your choice.

- Just eat the steak with asparagus, broccoli, cabbage, cauliflower, and Feta cheese on the side. Any meat or fish that's grilled or roasted is good for you.

- Juices, milkshakes, and sodas are off the table. Drink plenty of water, and order your tea or coffee with only heavy cream.

Lastly, at the end of it all, don't forget to ring the bell and say, "Yeeto!" if you are still on keto despite having eaten out.

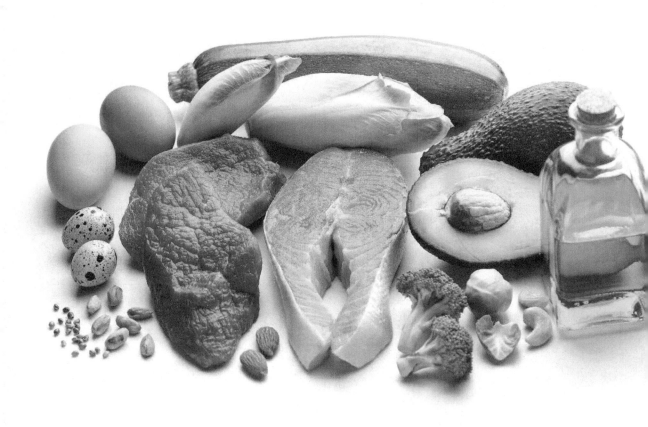

Chapter 13:
Pantry Essentials for Keto

I think shopping is truly the best retail therapy. If you agree, raise your hand and give a happy "Yeeto!" for keto. Now, let's go shopping for some pantry essentials. This is my most favorite part, right before the cooking and eating and, of course, seeing those fats melt away.

Anything that is extremely low in carbs is what you want to put in your shopping cart first. Do not even look at those whole grains. They aren't your friends when on keto, and most vegetables and fruits are not for you either. So what do you really get to buy? There's still a wide variety of delicious condiments and ingredients waiting for you to add to your pantry, so don't worry! With a little bit of guidance, you will also know where and how you can find them.

Being systematic and methodical is everything. The more organized you are, the easier your keto journey will be, so let me begin with giving you a pantry list of essentials first before you head out. These are everyday, basic items that you will need to have in order to quickly and easily whip up a yummy keto meal. These should give you a great head start into cooking for keto.

The Top Pantry Essentials

Arranged in the order of importance is the list of items that are great sources of the macros for you. Stocking up on some keto snacks is important—nuts and seeds are approved keto-friendly snacks. Avocado or hard-boiled eggs can be handy. In case of an emergency or if you are unable to cook for any reason, you won't have to go hungry or worse—eat food that's not keto-friendly.

There are some great spices and condiments on the list as well that will help you raise the flavor quotient of your meals. While you shop for the keto essentials listed out for you, see that you pick up unsweetened goods. Some people are okay with using artificial sweeteners to replace natural sugars in their keto cooking and baking. I will try and convince you not to because you don't actually need it. However, what you do need is salt.

During ketosis, your body is losing a lot of sodium, which is also the cause of side effects like light-headedness. It is, therefore, quite beneficial for you to add some salt to your foods.

Ketogenic diet specialists recommend 2,000-4,000 mg a day. Minimum daily sodium concentration (RDA) for regular diets is 2,300 mg. There are some fabulous salts to choose like the pink Himalayan salt, also called black salt, which is filled with minerals such as potassium, magnesium, and calcium (Wellversed Health, 2020). Then, there is always sea salt, rock salt, and even smoked salts for you to try. See what suits your taste the best.

While keto is all about high-fat foods, don't forget to add anti-inflammatory omega-3 fatty acids, particularly EPA and DHA, largely available in seafood. If you are not a pescatarian, then you could include it in your diet by taking a spoonful of cod liver oil or krill oil which are rich sources of the essential nutrients.

Fabulous Fat Sources

Apple Cider Vinegar	Almond Milk	Avocado	Avocado Oil / Avocado Oil Spray
Algae Oil—neutral-tasting oil for high-heat cooking	Balsamic Vinegar	Butter—preferably unsalted	Cacao Butter
Cheese—cheddar, blue cheese, Emmental, Feta, Gouda, mozzarella, Parmesan, provolone, etc.	Canola Oil	Coconut—dried/grated/desiccated	Coconut Milk
Coconut Oil	Cod Liver Oil	Cream—heavy/sour	Cream Cheese
Extra-Virgin Olive Oil	Flax Oil	Ghee	Krill Oil
Mayonnaise	MCT Oil	Nuts—almonds, cashews, hazelnuts, macadamia, pecan, peanuts, walnuts, etc.	Olives—black, green
Seeds—flax, pumpkin, sesame, sunflower, etc.	Sesame Oil	Sour Cream	Sugar-Free Dark Chocolate—90 % cacao or higher
White Vinegar			

Pro Protein Sources

Bacon	Beef—fatty cut steaks, ground, jerky, meat sticks, ribs, roast, etc.	Bratwurst	Chia Seeds
Chicken	Cheese	Duck	Eggs
Fish—fresh/canned mackerel, sardines, salmon, tuna, etc.	Goose	Greek Yogurt	Ham
Kale	Legumes	Mushrooms	Pepperoni
Peanut Butter	Pork Rinds	Quail	Salami
Sausages	Shellfish—crab, mussels, scallops, shrimp, oysters, squids, lobster, etc.	Spinach	Squash
Turkey	Veal		

Trusted Carb Sources

Artichokes	Asparagus	Bell Peppers—red, yellow, green	Berries—blackberries, blueberries, cranberries, raspberries, strawberries, etc.
Broccoli	Brussels Sprouts	Buckwheat	Cabbage
Cauliflower	Carrots	Celery	Cherry Tomatoes
Eggplant	Garlic	Green Beans	Leeks
Limes	Lemons	Lettuce	Okra
Radishes	Rhubarb	Small Baking Pumpkins	Spinach
Spring Onions	Shallots	Squash	Plum Tomatoes
Zucchini			

Keto-Friendly Baking Flours

Low-carb, keto-friendly flours are pantry essentials for those who love to bake and eat baked goods. Substitute the regular baking flours and make all the muffins, cakes, breads, and pancakes you like.

Almond Flour	Almond Meal or Ground Almonds	Coconut Flour
Ground Flax Meal	Psyllium Husk	Baking Powder

Spices and Condiments

What is food without the spices in the marinades or seasonings liberally sprinkled on top? Sauces and chutneys elevate the flavors on your plate instantly. What is baking without those extra aromatic flavorings? Traditional pickles and certain other probiotics are already known to you which you may safely include in your keto pantry.

Dried Herbs and Spices

Allspice	Black Pepper—whole/ground	Basil—dried	Caraway Seed
Cardamom—whole/powder	Cayenne Pepper	Chili Powder	Chili Flakes
Cinnamon—whole/powder	Cloves	Coriander Seeds—whole/powder	Cumin Seeds—whole/powder
Curry Leaves	Fennel Seeds—whole	Garlic Powder	Garam Masala (Indian Spice Blend)—whole/powder
Ginger—whole / ground paste / dried powder	Mace—whole/powder	Mustard Seeds—whole / powder / ground paste	Nutmeg—whole/powder
Onion Powder	Onion Seeds	Oregano	Paprika
Parsley—dried	Poppy Seeds	Pumpkin Pie Spice	Rosemary—dried
Szechuan Peppercorns	Turmeric Powder	Thyme—dried	

Condiments and Flavorings

Fresh Herbs—basil, chives, cilantro, coriander, dill, mint, parsley, etc.	Capers	Dill Pickle Relish
Horseradish Mustard	Lemon or Lime Juice	Mayonnaise
Mustard	Soy Sauce	Salsa
Peppermint Extract	Pumpkin Seeds—dried and salted	Pesto
Hot Sauce	Ketchup	Vanilla Extract

Now that you have a fairly comprehensive list of items that you can stock for your keto kitchen, you're probably eager to go shopping. I think Amazon is the best and most convenient way of getting most of the keto-friendly snacks, supplements, flours, condiments, and spices. If you like browsing the aisles, then you could go to your nearest Costco, Target, Trader Joe's, Walmart, or Whole Foods Market. And if you like to touch and smell the fresh produce before you buy, then you can locate a trusted local superstore, grocery store, or market for locally sourced items such as produce, grass-fed meats, seafood, green vegetables, etc.

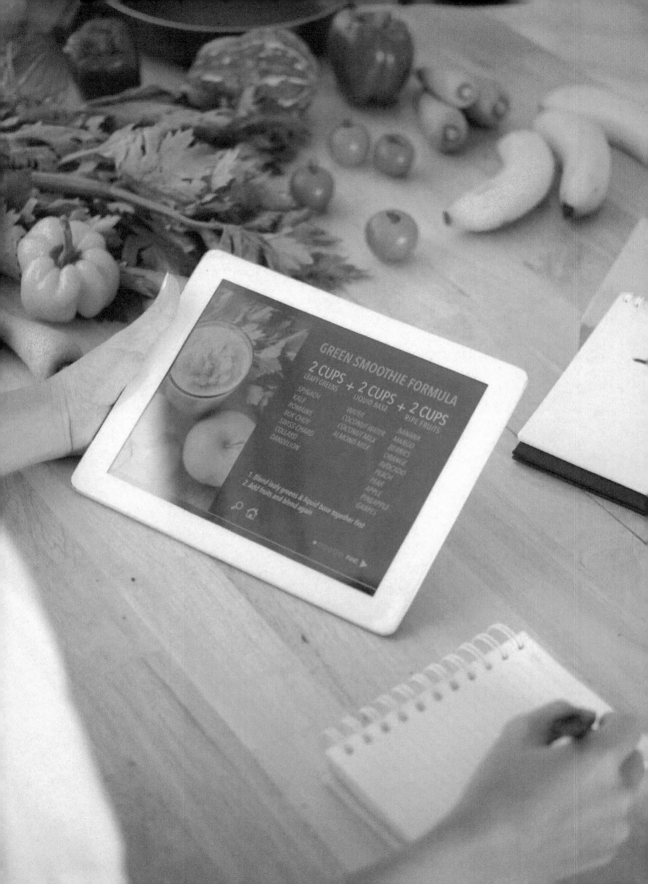

Chapter 14:
Refer to Simple, Quick-Prep Keto Recipes and Presto!

So you want to eat healthier, but you dread the idea of spending hours in the kitchen every week, don't you? It's pretty natural. Most people do not have the time, energy, or know-how to cook healthy meals. A keto life calls for healthy eating, and you know that. Yet I still never seem to see any reason to worry because keto cooking can be simpler than you think.

Just refer to the simple and quick-prep keto recipes that I have for you, and presto! You are on a roll!

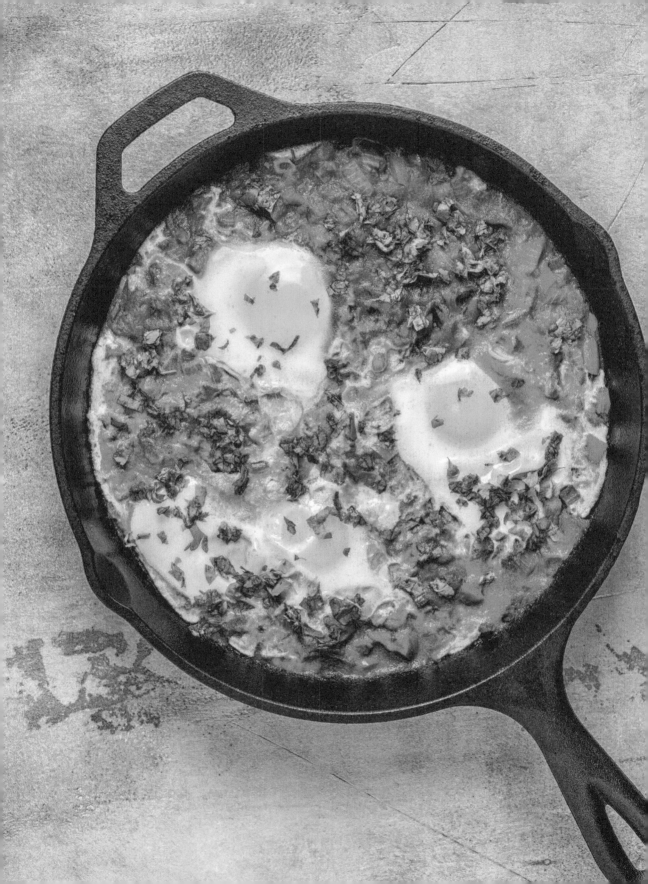

BREAKFAST IDEAS

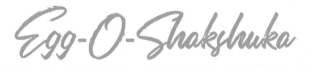

Egg-O-Shakshuka

Total Cooking Time:	Servings:	Calories/Serving:
20 minutes	1	274 cals

Estimated Keto Macros/Serving:		
Carbs:	Protein:	Fat:
3 grams	16 grams	22 grams

Originally a Middle Eastern recipe, this versatile low-carb keto dish needs only a few basic ingredients. Eggs get poached, so it is even healthier. You could even use only one skillet to prepare it, so you have less washing to do later, too.

Ingredients:

- 2 large eggs
- 1 tbsp unsalted butter
- 1 tsp extra-virgin olive oil
- 1 medium plum tomato, finely chopped
- 1 red bell pepper, finely chopped after removing the seeds and pith
- ½ onion, finely chopped
- 1 garlic clove, crushed
- 1.7 oz (50 g) crumbled Feta cheese
- 3.5 oz (100 g) fresh spinach, chopped
- 1 small bunch fresh coriander leaves, finely chopped for garnishing

Spices (to amp up the flavors):

- ¼ tsp paprika powder
- ¼ tsp cumin powder
- ¼ tsp coriander powder
- ¼ tsp turmeric powder
- Pinch of ground black pepper
- Pinch of chili flakes
- Salt to taste

Directions:

1. Place the skillet on the top of the stove over medium flame.

2. Add the butter to the skillet and let it melt.

3. Add the chopped onions and crushed garlic and let cook together for 3 minutes until the onions turn slightly pink and translucent. Don't let them brown.

4. Add the chopped tomatoes and cover the skillet to let them sweat for 3 minutes. I like to sprinkle some salt in at this stage so that the sauce base tastes great, too.

5. Except for the pepper and chili flakes, add all the spice powders and give it a nice stir so it becomes a healthy mixture.

6. Add the bell peppers and spinach at this stage. Slowly add ½ cup water to let the veggies cook together with the sauce. Cover and cook for 3-5 minutes.

7. Take a spoon and create two wells in the sauce.

8. Crack one egg each into each well. Take care to see that the yellow yolk remains intact as you drop it in. Let the egg whites spread around the well. I like to sprinkle some salt and pepper over the eggs at this stage.

9. Cover and cook for another 2-3 minutes until you see the egg whites are fairly cooked, but be sure to keep the yolks slightly runny.

10. Switch off the flame and take the skillet off the cooktop.

11. Spread the crumbled Feta cheese all over.

12. Garnish it with coriander leaves.

13. You could drizzle the extra-virgin olive oil at the edges of the skillet and around the eggs.

14. Enjoy your meal while it's still warm.

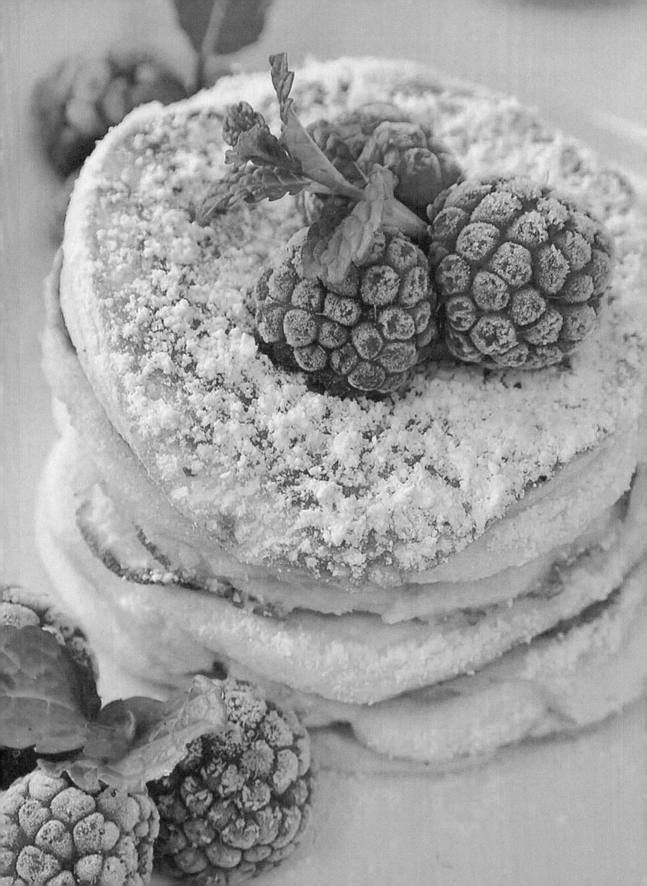

Yeeto Keto Pancakes

Total Cooking Time:	Servings:	Calories/Serving:
20 minutes	1 (5 small pancakes)	55 cals

Estimated Keto Macros/Serving:		
Carbs:	Protein:	Fat:
3.3 grams	4.3 grams	10.7 grams

I need fluffy pancakes for breakfast at least once a week... period.

Ingredients:

- 1 large egg
- 1 tbsp butter
- 1 tbsp avocado oil
- ¼ cup almond milk
- ½ cup super-fine almond flour (not the almond meal)
- ½ tsp vanilla extract
- ½ tsp cinnamon powder
- ½ tsp baking powder
- Salt to taste

Directions:

1. Combine the ingredients and prepare the batter in a big bowl if you are adept at manually doing it. If you have access to an electric mixer, that's perfect! If you are using a traditional blender, that works too!

2. So in goes the almond milk, the egg, the avocado oil, and vanilla extract first. Blend it quickly but make sure you beat the egg well.

3. Next, add all of the other ingredients: almond flour, cinnamon, baking powder, and salt.

4. Blend the mixture until it has formed a pretty smooth batter of pouring consistency. If mixing manually, make sure that there are no lumps or air bubbles trapped in the batter.

5. I usually let the batter sit happily for five minutes.

6. Meanwhile, heat a skillet on the stovetop over a medium flame and melt a little butter in it. Do not let it burn. I usually pour one ladleful of the batter and lightly spread it to make small pancakes.

7. It's fun to watch it cook as bubbles start popping on the surface and the pancake begins to rise. You will know it's cooked when the edges are set and can be turned up easily with the spatula.

8. Here we go! Now comes the fun part: Flip the pancake over and let it cook through on the other side.

9. It takes about 3–4 minutes for each side to turn golden brown.

10. Flip the skillet carefully to take the pancake off on a plate, or skip the antics and simply use a spatula.

11. Grease the skillet once again and start all over to make four more fluffy pancakes.

12. Enjoy your delicious breakfast.

13. For the final touch, you can enjoy your pancakes with store-bought, sugar-free, and keto-friendly maple syrup. Or try blueberry sauce instead. If you are lucky enough, you will find both of these items online.

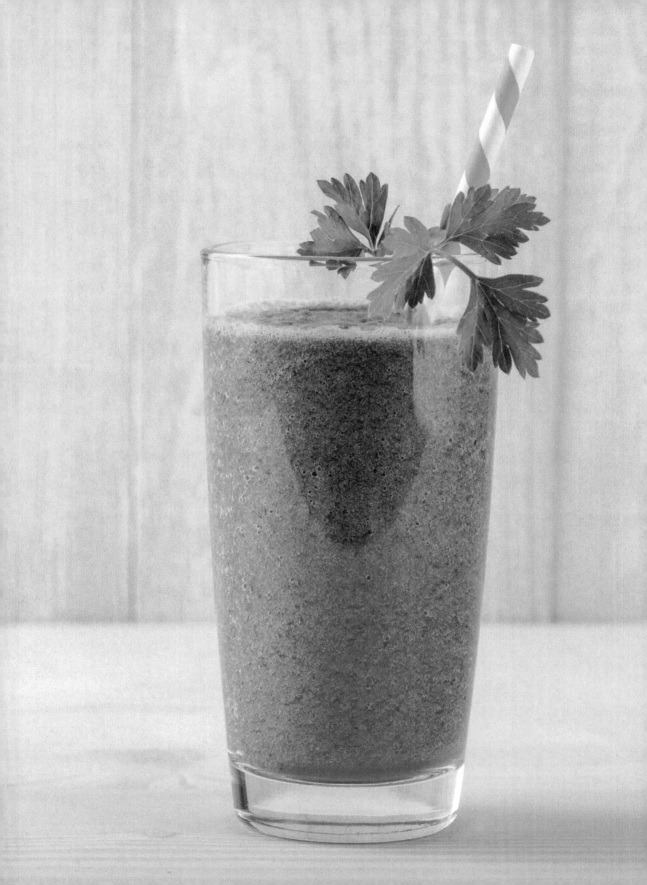

DRINKS AND SMOOTHIES

Very Berry Green Smoothie

Total Cooking Time:	Servings:	Calories/Serving:
5 minutes	1	90 cals

Estimated Keto Macros/Serving:		
Carbs:	Protein:	Fat:
11 grams	2 grams	19 grams

You will be surprised to learn that kale is neutral to taste, hence, it's a great way to bulk up your smoothie with a great source of vitamins. And this smoothie just might taste like liquid cheesecake... seriously!

Ingredients:

- ¼ avocado, chopped and peeled
- ½ cup kale
- 1 tbsp coconut oil
- ½ lemon with juice extracted
- 1 tsp fresh ginger root
- 10 frozen blueberries
- ½ cup frozen strawberries, sliced

Directions:

1. Preparing this smoothie is a no-brainer. You simply drop one ingredient after another into the blender and then, "Yeeto!" You've got yourself a low-carb, high-on-taste breakfast smoothie. If it's too thick in consistency, you can thin it with a little water if you like.
2. Oh, and don't forget: Enjoy good health!

Pro Tip: I wouldn't add any artificial sweetener because the berries bring their own natural flavors, but if you must, use one or two drops of liquid stevia sweetener.

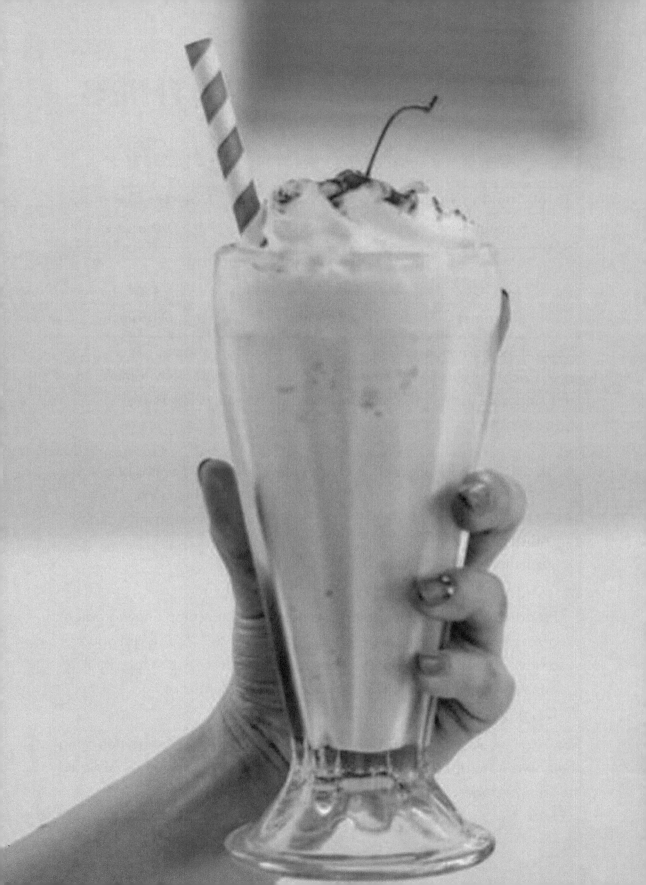

Peppermint-O Milkshake

Total Cooking Time:	Servings:	Calories/Serving:
5 minutes	1	165 cals

Estimated Keto Macros/Serving:		
Carbs:	Protein:	Fat:
2 grams	2 grams	17 grams

The definition of milky white goodness, this milkshake is sure to remind you of snow and maybe Christmas, too.

Ingredients:

➢ ¾ cup almond milk

➢ 1 cup vanilla ice cream, low-carb and sugar-free

➢ ½ tsp peppermint extract

➢ 2 tbsp heavy cream, whipped

➢ Sprinkles, optional (but you know you'll want them!)

Directions:

1. Again, preparing this milkshake requires no special skills. Just put the almond milk, ice cream, and peppermint extract in your trusty blender and blend away for a minute or two until you feel it's smooth.

2. Pour the shake mix into a glass.

3. Top it up with the heavy whipped cream and sprinkles.

4. Sip it up and start your keto day with some "Yeeto!"

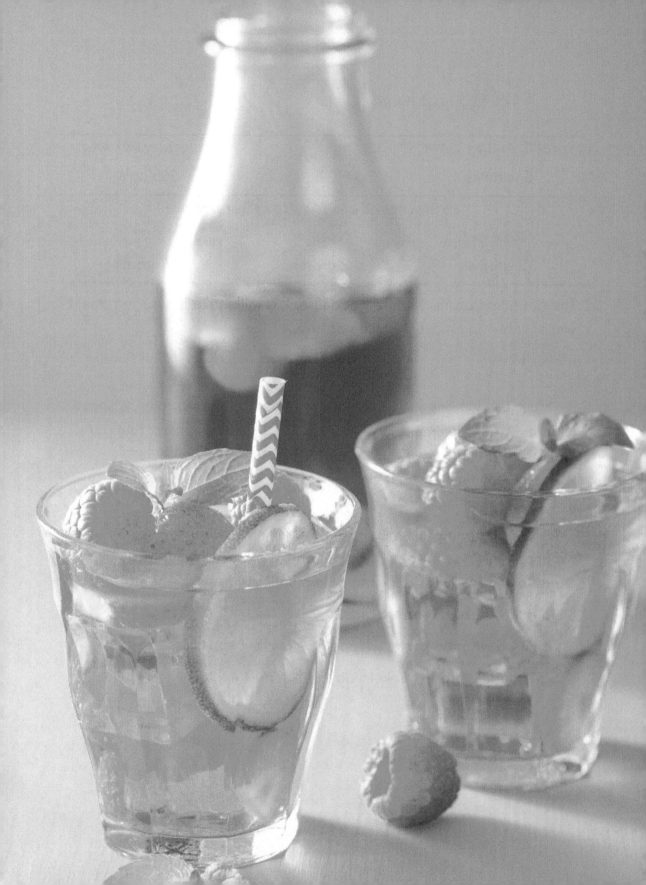

Berry Lime-O-Made

Total Cooking Time:	Servings:	Calories/Serving:
30 minutes	5	7 cals

Estimated Keto Macros/Serving:		
Carbs:	**Protein:**	**Fat:**
3 grams	0.2 grams	0 grams

This is a refreshing, low-carb drink that will clean your palate and act as a cooling refreshment on those hot summer days.

Ingredients:

- 5.2 oz (150 g) mixed frozen berries: blueberries, blackberries, black currants, cherries, strawberries, and/or raspberries
- 1 big lime or 2 lemons with the juice extracted
- 1 bunch of fresh mint leaves
- 33 fl oz (1 liter) water (You'll need lots!)
- Ice cubes to make it a nice and chilled drink.
- 10-15 drops of liquid stevia or any low-carb artificial sweetener, if you want to add some sweetness to this concoction.

Directions:

1. Once again, easy-yeety lemon-squeezy—literally!
2. Take a big punch bowl and drop in your berry mix.
3. Squeeze out the lime/lemon juice over the berries.
4. Lightly peel the rind of the lime/lemons so that it does not make the drink bitter. Thinly slice it up, and drop it in, too.
5. Pour in the water, and add the artificial sweetener.
6. Refrigerate before drinking if you like it well- chilled. Let the water infuse for 25-30 minutes. The longer you let it stand, the more flavorsome the drink will be.
7. Serve and add ice cubes to the glass. I like lots of them in mine! Cheers!

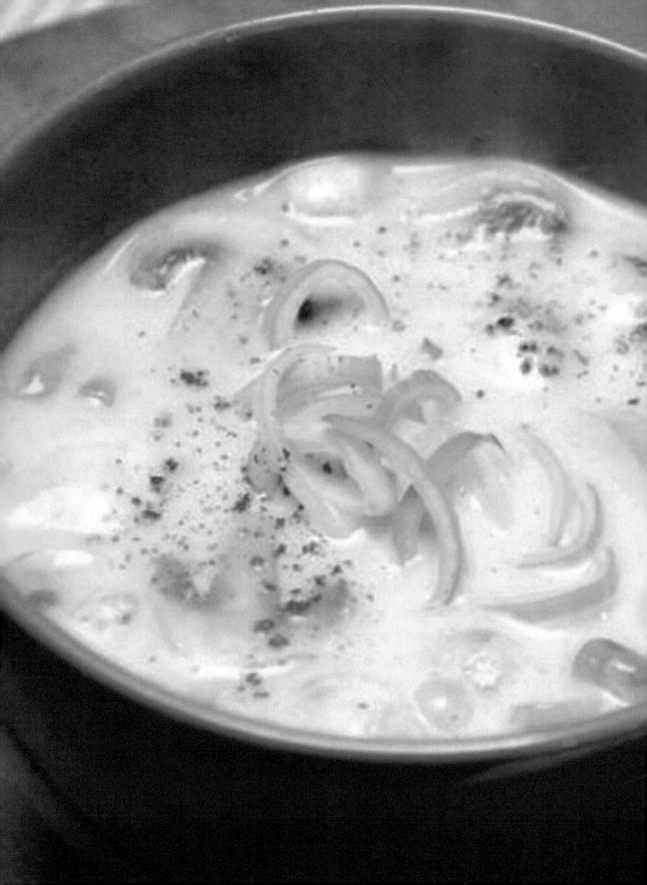

SOUPS AND SALADS

Cream-O-Mushroom Soup

Total Cooking Time:	Servings:	Calories/Serving:
30 minutes	4	379 cals

Estimated Keto Macros/Serving:		
Carbs:	Protein:	Fat:
15 grams	11 grams	33 grams

This is one of the soups that I call soul food. It can warm up the cockles of your mushy heart!

Ingredients:

- 1 pound (500 g) fresh button mushrooms, sliced
- 2 tbsp butter
- 1 medium onion, finely chopped
- 2 cloves garlic, crushed
- 5 cups chicken stock
- 4 oz (113 g) cream cheese
- ¾ cup heavy cream
- ½ tsp ground black pepper
- Small bunch of parsley, finely chopped for garnishing
- Fresh thyme for garnishing
- Salt to taste

Directions:

1. Place a medium-sized soup pot on the top of the stove and set heat to medium.

2. Melt the butter, add the crushed garlic, and then add the chopped onions into the pot.

3. Cover and cook the onions for about 4-5 minutes until they have turned slightly pink and translucent, and the aroma of the garlic is wafting. Some love to caramelize the onions for more flavor. That's cool, but make sure you don't burn them.

4. Meanwhile, you can clean and slice the mushrooms. Hold each mushroom sideways, head up and tail down. Then, slice to get neat, T-shaped pieces.

5. Add all the mushrooms to the onions and let them sweat out all the water. You will see them shrivel and brown. This may take about 5 minutes. Do not let them burn. I like to add some salt and stir everything well at this stage.

6. Save ½ cup of the chicken stock for the creamy sauce and pour the rest into the soup pot. Add thyme and stir well. Bring the pot to a boil.

7. Cover and let pot simmer on low for about 10 minutes.

8. In the meantime, prepare the cream sauce in a blender. Blend the remaining chicken stock with cream cheese at top speed to get a smooth, purée-like consistency.

9. Add the blended cream along with the heavy cream to the soup pot and stir. Over a medium flame, the pot will begin to boil again after about 2-3 minutes. Season with salt and pepper at this stage.

10. Lower the flame and let it simmer. You might have to keep stirring the pot from time to time for 5 minutes or so.

11. Take the pot off the flame, scoop out a serving, and enjoy some piping hot and creamy soup.

12. Garnish with finely chopped parsley and say "Yeeto!"

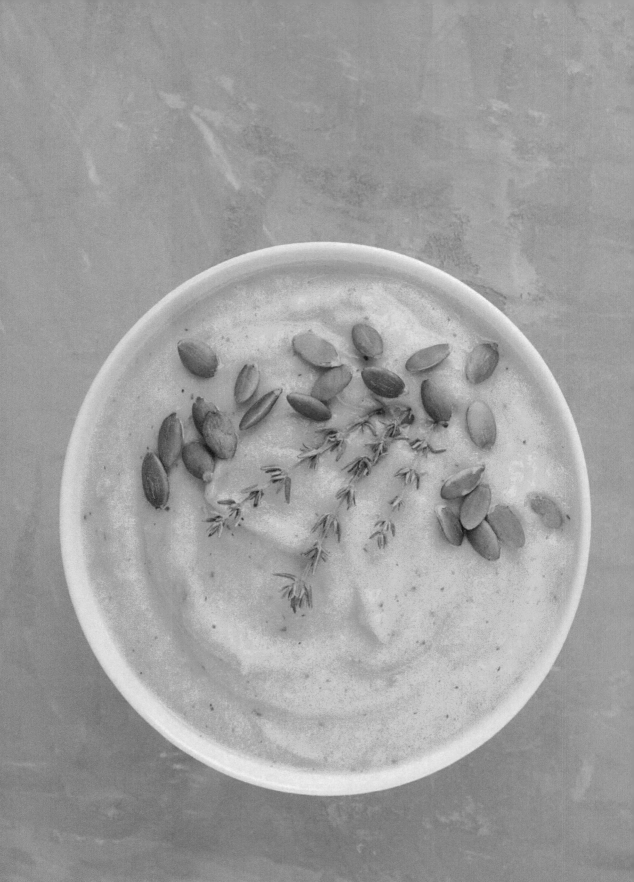

Phat Pumpkin Soup

Total Cooking Time:	Servings:	Calories/Serving:
30 minutes	4	190 cals

Estimated Keto Macros/Serving:		
Carbs:	Protein:	Fat:
10 grams	7 grams	11 grams

Fall or winter, keto or not, pumpkin soup will never go out of style!

Ingredients:

- 17 oz (500 g) pumpkin purée
- 4 cups of vegetable stock
- ½ tsp garlic powder
- ¼ tsp red chili flakes
- ½ cup heavy cream
- ¼ cup sour cream for garnishing—optional
- 2 tbsp pumpkin seeds, roasted and salted for garnishing—optional
- ½ tsp black pepper
- 1 tsp dried thyme for garnishing
- Salt to taste

Directions:

1. Place the soup pot on top of the stove and set to medium heat.

2. Except for the creams, add all the listed ingredients to the pot one after another.

3. Stir and mix it all well. Cover and cook for about 10 minutes.

4. Bring the pot to a boil and then let it simmer on low flame for about 5 minutes.

5. Remove pot from the heat. Let the steam exit, and then mix in the heavy cream.

6. Salt and add more pepper if you like, to taste.

7. When you are ready to eat, ladle this creamy soup into a bowl and garnish it with sour cream and those crunchy, salty roasted pumpkin seeds. Bon appétit!

Pro Tip: Use small baking pumpkins to make a silky smooth purée. Remove the seeds and roast in an oven for about 30 minutes with the peel. Take out the softened center and purée pumpkins in a blender. It's very easy to make, plus the added benefit of the sweet phat aroma that will waft through your home. Short on time? You can also use canned purée to reduce the preparation time.

Save the pumpkin seeds to roast and salt them. They work well as a keto snack.

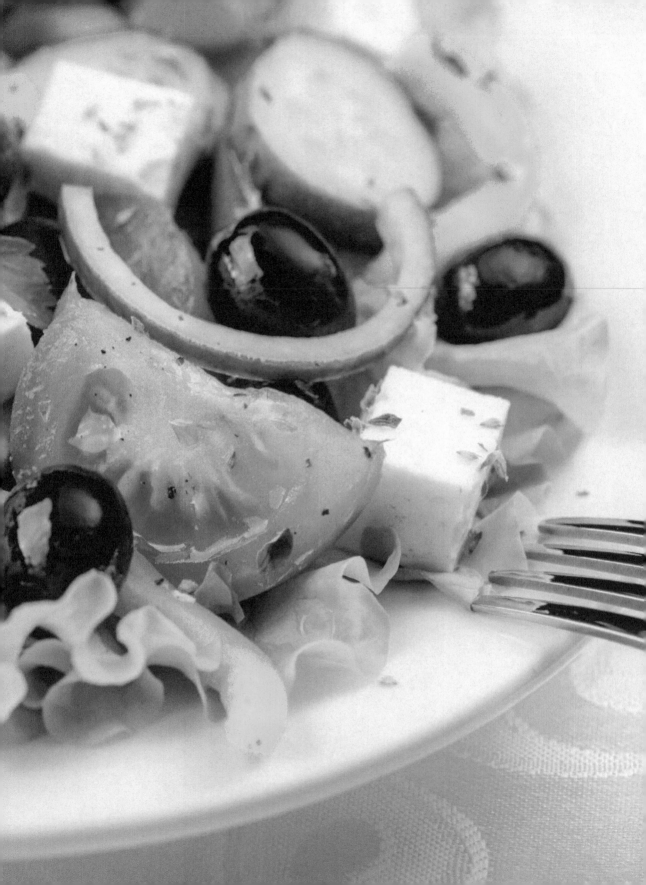

Green Greek Salad

Total Cooking Time:	Servings:	Calories/Serving:
10 minutes	1	60 cals

Estimated Keto Macros/Serving:		
Carbs:	**Protein:**	**Fat:**
3 grams	5 grams	2 grams

Make yourself a delicious bowl of this historical Horiatiki salad with a contemporary keto twist.

Ingredients:

- 1 small cucumber, peeled and diced
- 1 ½ big ripe plum tomatoes, diced (or) 5 oz (150 g) cherry tomatoes, halved
- ¼ red or yellow bell pepper, diced

- ¼ green bell pepper, diced
- 1 small zucchini, sliced
- ¼ red onion, thinly sliced
- 8 to 10 black olives, pitted and sliced
- 3.5 oz (100 g) Feta cheese, crumbled

For the Vinaigrette:

- ¼ tbsp red wine vinegar
- 3 tbsp extra-virgin olive oil
- Pinch of dried oregano
- Pinch of chili flakes

- Pinch of black pepper
- 1 clove garlic, finely minced
- Salt to taste

Directions:

1. Except for cleaning and chopping the vegetables, there's not really much to do for prep!

2. Next, take a large salad bowl and bring all the veggies together in it.

3. In a small bowl, make a vinaigrette salad dressing by combining all the ingredients separately, then mix.

4. Drizzle vinaigrette over your salad bowl.

5. Salt and pepper to taste.

6. Crumble some Feta cheese over the salad.

7. Voila! It's ready for you to chow down on this yummy, healthy green bowl and say "Yeeto!"

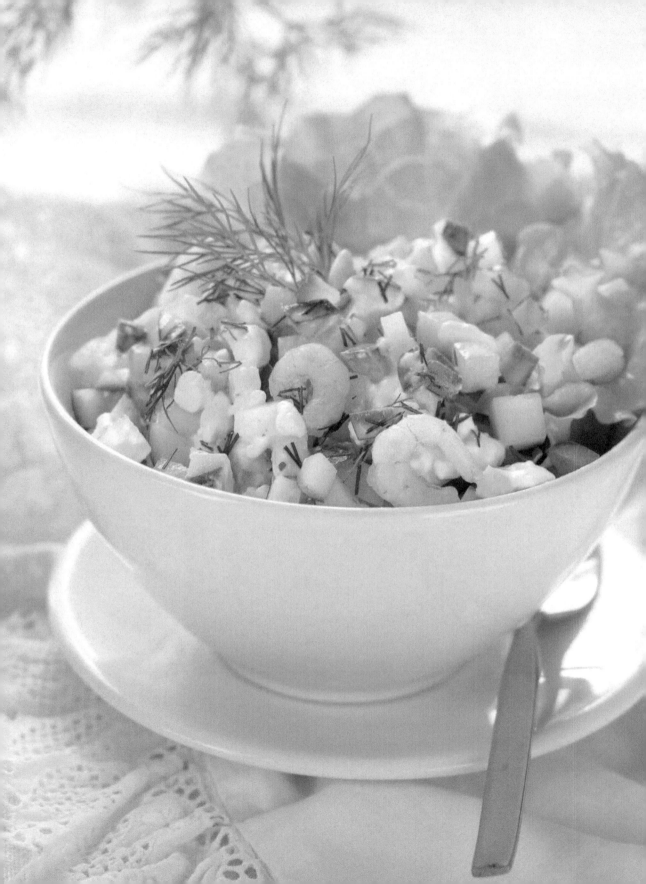

Shrimpy-O Salad

Total Cooking Time:	Servings:	Calories/Serving:
10 minutes	4	134 cals

Estimated Keto Macros/Serving:		
Carbs:	Protein:	Fat:
4 grams	20 grams	5 grams

A salivate-at-sight plate for seafood lovers. It's not just the tummy that's going to feel satiated. Your taste buds have a "Yeeto!" treat coming. Plus, this is so easy to whip up.

Ingredients:

- ⅓ cup sour cream
- 1 pound (500 g) small fresh shrimps peeled and deveined. You can also use thawed frozen shrimp here, too.
- 1 tbsp extra-virgin olive oil
- 2 tbsp butter, unsalted
- 2 clove garlic, minced
- ½ cup celery, finely chopped
- ½ cup cucumber, finely chopped
- 1 big onion, finely chopped
- 2 tbsp lemon juice
- ¼ tsp red chili flakes
- ¼ tsp black pepper
- ¼ tsp red paprika
- Bunch of fresh dill, chopped for garnishing
- Salt to taste

Directions:

1. Take a large salad bowl and whisk the sour cream until it's smooth.

2. Add a tablespoon of the lemon juice, red chili flakes, black pepper, and a pinch of salt to the bowl and whisk everything together.

3. Place a medium-sized pan on the top of the stove over medium flame and melt the butter.

4. Swirl it all around the pan before adding the shrimp and minced garlic to it.

5. Quickly drizzle ½ tablespoon of the lemon juice over the cooking shrimp and sprinkle red paprika, some dill, and a pinch of salt, too.

6. Let it cook in the lemon-butter sauce, but not for too long. Fresh shrimp won't take more than 4 or 5 minutes to cook thoroughly. Thawed frozen shrimp will also cook quickly. Toss the shrimp around and quickly move all the contents of the pan into the large salad bowl.

7. Add the chopped cucumber, celery, and onion to it, as well.

8. Mix everything well and drizzle olive oil over it.

9. Garnish with the remaining dill and serve.

10. Don't skimp on the shrimp. Throw your worries to the air and enjoy this healthy, low-carb salad!

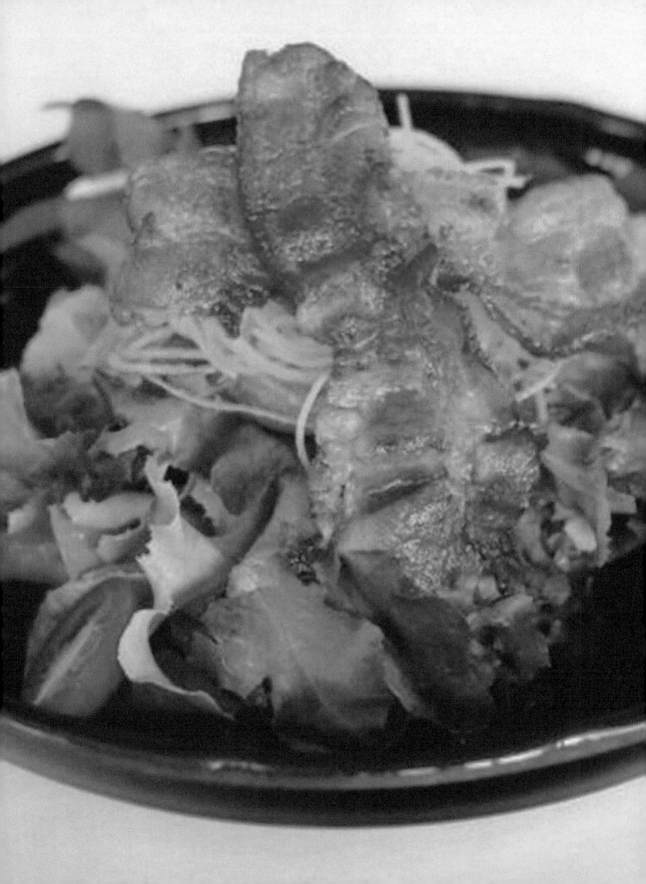

Hi-Low BLT Salad

Total Cooking Time:	Servings:	Calories/Serving:
10 minutes	6	202 cals

Estimated Keto Macros/Serving:		
Carbs:	Protein:	Fat:
6 grams	6.5 grams	17.5 grams

Flavor combinations are everything to make this simple dish taste oh-so-yeeto!

Ingredients:

➤ 6 smoked bacon strips

➤ 18 oz (500 g) iceberg lettuce

➤ 3 small plum tomatoes, diced (or) 5 oz (150 g) cherry tomatoes, halved

➤ ½ onion, thinly sliced

➤ ½ cup cheddar cheese, shredded

For the Salad Dressing:

➤ 6 tbsp mayonnaise

➤ Few sprigs of dill, finely chopped

➤ 3 tbsp sour cream

➤ 1 tsp garlic powder

➤ ½ tsp dried parsley

➤ ½ tsp paprika

➤ ½ tbsp apple cider vinegar

➤ Salt to taste

Directions:

1. Put a frying pan on the top of the stove over a medium flame and place the bacon strips in it neatly in a row. You do not need to add butter or oil to the pan. Bacon will release its own juices and cook in its own fats.

2. Meanwhile, in a large salad bowl, combine the iceberg lettuce, cherry tomatoes, and onions.

3. In another smaller bowl, mix in all the ingredients listed for the salad dressing. You could add some tablespoons of water to get the desired consistency.

4. Once the bacon strips are cooked evenly, take them out of the pan and chop them into smaller bite-sized pieces. Add them to the salad bowl and mix everything well.

5. Now serve one helping in a bowl. Sprinkle shredded cheddar cheese and layer the salad dressing on top.

6. At every sumptuous mouthful, you are sure to be surprised, what you are enjoying is a "Hi" on taste but "Low" on carbs keto meal.

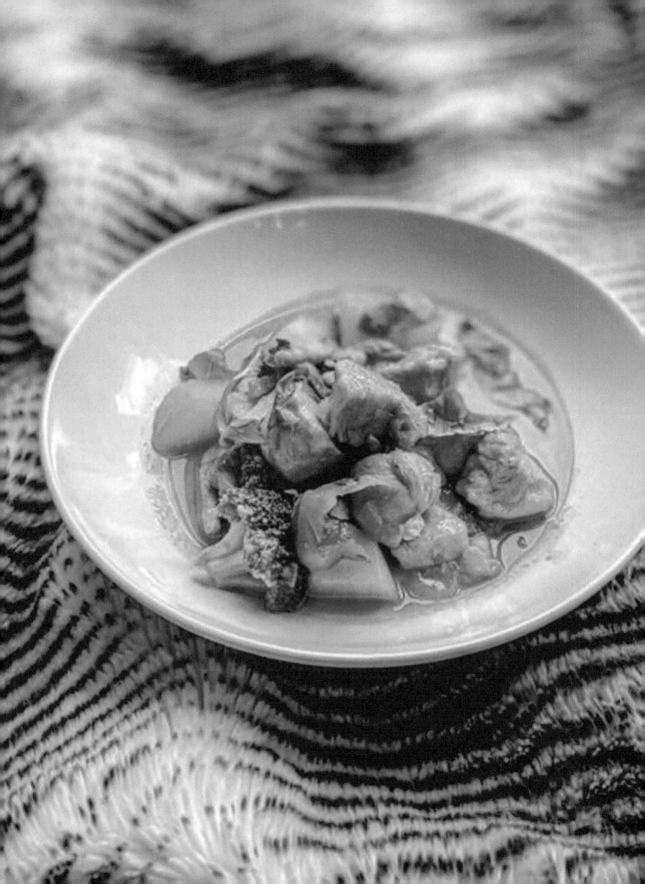

MAIN DISHES

Pro-Keto Chicken Stew with Cauliflower Rice

Total Cooking Time: 50 minutes	Servings: 6	Calories/Serving: 196 cals in the chicken stew, 98 kcals in the cauliflower rice

Chicken Stew Estimated Keto Macros/Serving:		
Carbs:	Protein:	Fat:
6 grams	27 grams	10.5 grams

Cauliflower Rice Estimated Keto Macros/Serving:		
Carbs:	Protein:	Fat:
7 grams	0 grams	7 grams

Some dishes make me long for rice to go with it. Does that happen to you, too? So let me tell you that cauliflower rice just makes a heavenly pairing with this stew. Try it!

Ingredients:

- 1 pound (500 g) fresh chicken (boneless thighs), cubed. Alternatively, you could also use frozen chicken breasts and thaw then chop them into cubes.
- 1 large head of cauliflower, cleaned and cut into florets
- 3 tbsp avocado oil
- 2 stalks celery, finely chopped
- 2 large onions, finely chopped
- 5 or 6 cloves garlic, minced
- 1 big lemon for juice extract
- 1 tsp black pepper
- ½ tsp dried thyme leaves
- Small bunch of coriander leaves, finely chopped

- ➤ Small bunch of cilantro leaves, finely chopped
- ➤ ½ tsp paprika
- ➤ 4 cups of chicken broth
- ➤ Salt to taste

Directions For Chicken Stew:

1. Pick a heavy-bottomed pot to make a substantial quantity of the stew and place it over medium heat on the top of the stove.

2. Add the avocado oil to the pot and, over it, add the chopped onions.

3. I like to add the minced garlic to the onions right about now because the mixed aroma of onions and garlic cooking together is just divine.

4. Cover and cook for 4 or 5 minutes until the onions have turned slightly pink and translucent, and the raw smell of the garlic is gone.

5. Add the paprika seasoning first, followed by the finely chopped celery, and then give it a good mix. I like to sprinkle some salt at this stage and pepper the mix, too.

6. Add the boneless chicken pieces in and sauté everything by adding a little more avocado oil to the pot. This will not only lock in the flavors of the meat but also make it juicy and tender on the inside. Don't fry the chicken on high flame.

7. Add the chicken broth and thyme, and let the pot boil.

8. Squeeze in the juice of half a lemon. Cover the pot with a lid and leave it to simmer on a low flame for 20-25 minutes. Even if it's frozen, thawed chicken, it does not need additional time to cook.

9. In the meantime, you could start preparing the cauliflower rice.

10. Once the stew has been simmering on the stove for around 20 to 25 minutes, switch off the flame and take the pot off the top of the stove.

11. Garnish the stew with chopped coriander, and it's ready to eat.

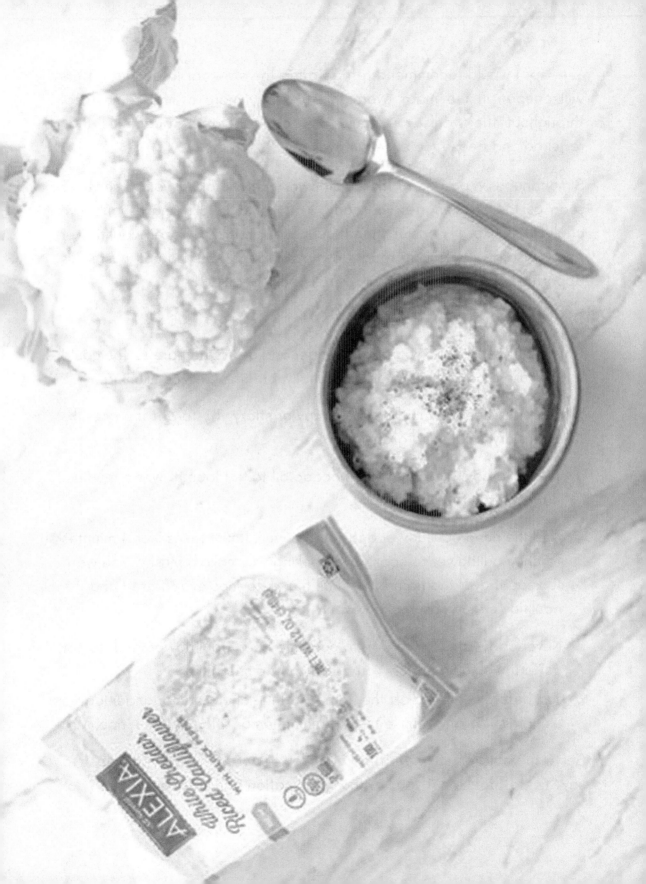

Pro Tip: I would recommend refrigerating the stew for later. The flavors will deepen in the meat overnight. To enjoy more of the same meal throughout the week, you could also cook in larger quantities than required and freeze the excess stew.

Simultaneously, preparing the cauliflower rice will allow you to serve as soon as the chicken stew is ready. You could quickly make your own cauliflower rice. It's easier than it sounds—I promise! Frozen cauliflower rice is also available as a ready-to-make product, but do not waste this opportunity for enhancing your overall cooking skills.

Directions for Cauliflower Rice:

1. Put all the florets in your food blender and grate the florets. You could also use a box grater to do it manually, but it is time-consuming.

2. The consistency should not be lumpy or sticky. Try to get the rice-like grains dry, small, and granular.

3. Take a large skillet and add avocado oil to it. Place it over a medium flame on the top of the stove.

4. Add the riced cauliflower and sauté it well. It just takes 3 or 4 minutes for the cauliflower to cook. Overcooking will make it mushy. You want to keep it over the flame only until the water has evaporated and the cauliflower rice has cooked evenly.

5. Never add water to the pan to cook the riced cauliflower, and do not cover it with a lid either. You don't want to steam it.

6. Just before switching off the flame, add the chopped coriander leaves as garnishing and drizzle the remaining lemon juice over the rice. Mix

Serve the chicken stew with the cauliflower rice. Oh, and remember to say "Yeeto!" for keto if you like the combination of mains as much as I do!

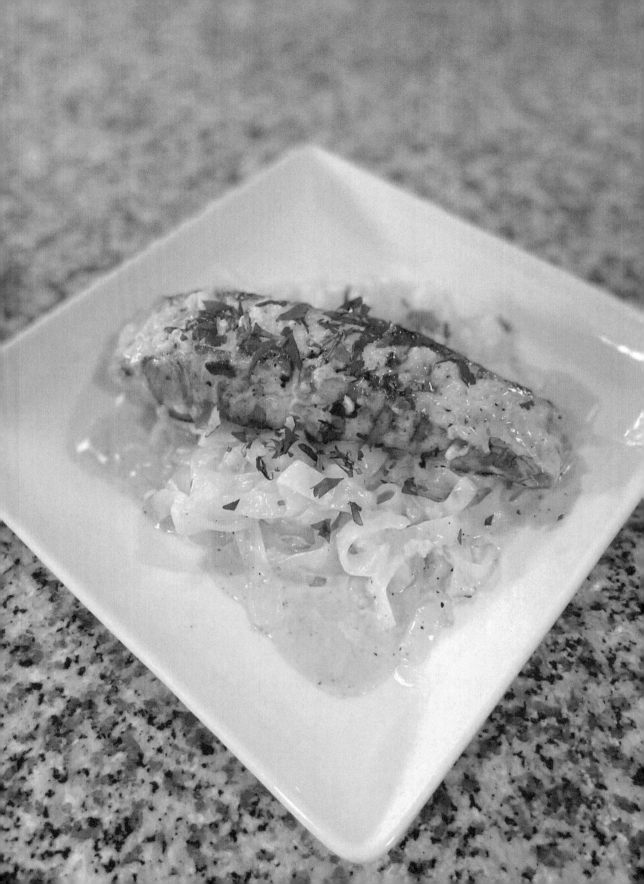

Creamy-O Salmon with Noodles

Total Cooking Time:	Servings:	Calories/Serving:
30 minutes	4	521 cals in the creamy salmon, 40 cals in the konjac noodles

Salmon Estimated Keto Macros/Serving:		
Carbs:	Protein:	Fat:
6 grams	29 grams	41 grams

Konjac (Shirataki) Estimated Keto Macros/Serving:		
Carbs:	Protein:	Fat:
8 grams	0 grams	0 grams

Salmon swim against the stream just like keto dieters who have a lot to struggle against until they get into the right zone. Even a meat lover will enjoy this, I bet. You can celebrate with a hearty "Yeeto!" for this keto recipe when you get to eat this delicious lemony, buttery salmon and still burn fat.

Ingredients:

- 4 salmon fillets of 4 oz (115 g) each, skin-on preferred
- 28 oz (800 g) of konjac noodles (or Shirataki noodles)
- 4 tbsp avocado oil
- 1 ¼ cup heavy cream
- ½ cup Parmesan cheese, grated
- 2 tbsp lemon juice
- 3 cloves garlic, minced
- Pinch of black pepper
- Small bunch of fresh parsley, chopped for garnishing
- Salt to taste

Directions for Creamy Salmon:

1. If you have a cast-iron skillet, there's nothing like it! Fry off all four fillets at once, so you save on time. Choose the skillet size accordingly.

2. Place the skillet on the top of the stove over medium heat and add the avocado oil to it.

3. Place the salmon fillets in the skillet, skin-side up and neatly in a row.

4. Do not try to flip the fillet before it is completely cooked, as you will break it. The first sign that it's cooked is when the corners at the bottom begin to turn and the fillet easily releases off the pan. It shouldn't take more than 3 or 4 minutes for a 4-oz fillet.

5. Flip the fillet with a good firm spatula and let the skin crisp up completely to a lovely golden-brown color.

6. Remove the fillets from the skillet, place them on a plate and let them rest.

7. To the same skillet that may still have a little oil left in it, add the minced garlic.

8. Add in the heavy cream and mix everything properly.

9. Sprinkle the black pepper into the pan and add salt to taste.

10. Let the sauce simmer on a low flame for 4-5 minutes until it thickens.

11. Switch off the flame and add the lemon juice and mix well.

12. Let the salmon swim in the lemon cream sauce when you serve and garnish your plate with parsley.

Pro Tip: Never put thawed-from-frozen salmon directly on the pan. Let it come back to room temperature and become evenly soft to touch. Pat it dry with paper towels. Rub the salt and pepper into the skin and fillet on all sides. Brush each fillet with some oil.

White juice releasing from the fillet is the first sign that it's been overcooked.

You could make it a wholesome plate by serving it with some silky konjac noodles. These Japanese noodles made from the root of the konjac plant are keto-friendly and extremely easy to make. They are known as miracle noodles for that very reason, I suppose.

Konjac noodles are easily available online on Amazon, or you will also find them in superstores that offer healthy foods. Alternatively, you can also use zucchini noodles ("zoodles") for an added twist!

You can prepare excess noodles and refrigerate for later. They are easy to reheat as well, but do not freeze them!

Directions for Konjac/Shirataki Noodles:

1. Using a colander, rinse the noodles in cold running water.
2. Drain and put them on a tray to pat them dry with paper napkins. The less water in them, the better and quicker they cook.
3. Take a medium-sized skillet and place it over medium flame. Do not add any oil.
4. Put the noodles in the pan and keep stirring them around. See that you do not break them to bits. Let the water evaporate.
5. It shouldn't take the noodles too long to cook. A maximum of 10 minutes will be fine. You will know once they appear really dry.
6. Switch off the flame and sprinkle the grated Parmesan on top and mix well.
7. The salmon in creamy sauce is waiting for the konjac noodles to be added to the plate.
8. Do that and see it become a happier meal. Enjoy!

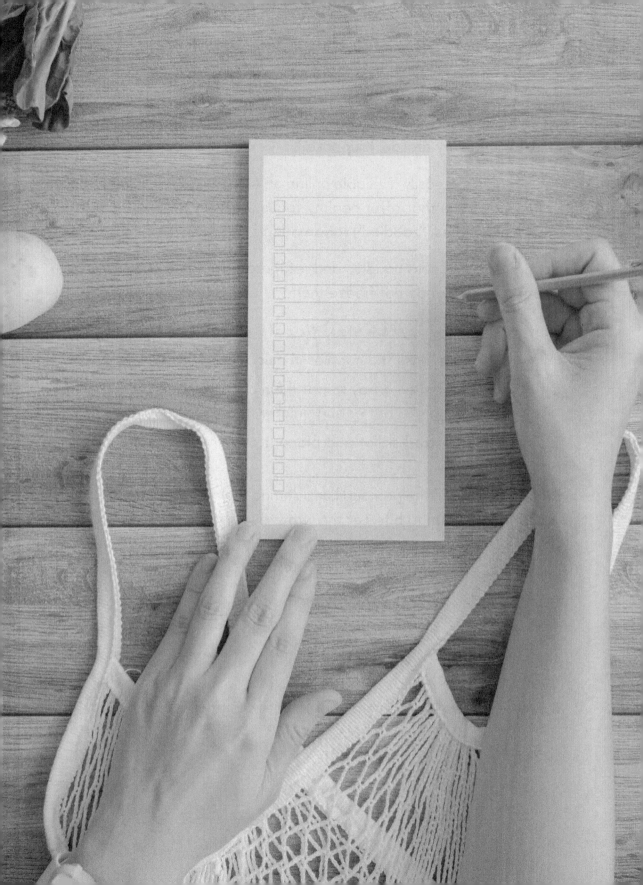

Chapter 15:
Sample Grocery List-O

The ketogenic diet might be a perennially trending buzzword between fitness enthusiasts, but at the end of the day, it's just an eating plan done right! So do not let yourself get overwhelmed by information overload.

At the risk of sounding repetitive, if you're trying to burn fat, you need to eat in a calorie deficit. Though all are made differently, a general assumption is that you should consume less than 2,000 calories per day to maintain ketosis. Please see your doctor or nutritionist before you start off, so your daily macros budget is clear to you.

To help you continue with conviction on your keto journey, here's a sample grocery list based on the quick-prep recipes given in this book. This should be on top of your to-do list. It can remain pinned to your refrigerator under your favorite fridge magnet, as this can be your go-to grocery shopping list for the next two weeks (and hopefully on a repeat to restock for the subsequent two weeks later).

Once you have restocked a few times down the line, you will get more confident and not need a list to guide you at all. You will have found out what works and doesn't for you as well as what you like and dislike. Then, you will shop from your healthy heart for your healthy gut, mind, and physique.

Two-Week Grocery List

Note that the grocery list is provided assuming that you are not eating alone, and you will be serving a minimum of four people. It's based on the recipes provided in the book, so you can start trying them out right away. Feel free to tweak the list and personalize it as per your choices—for, example, some may love eggs for breakfast every day, and some keto dieters are pure vegetarians.

The shopping list provided is a template to simply refer to and use to draw up your own. Sizes and measures may vary by brand.

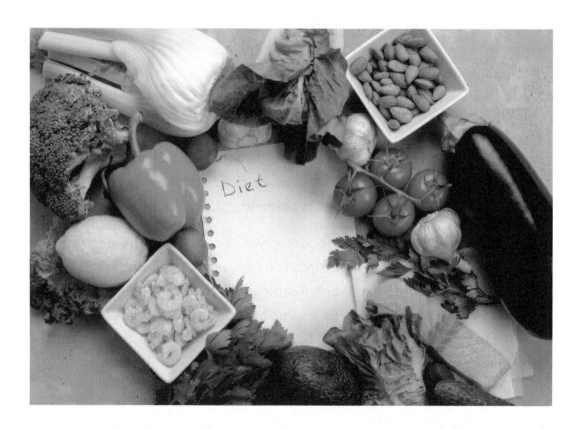

Week 1 Shopping List

Fresh Produce:

4 avocados	garlic bulb	2 red bell peppers
2 yellow bell peppers	2 green bell peppers	2 onions (one white and one red)
1 small bunch of green onions	½ pound of fresh button mushrooms	1 bunch of spinach
3 cucumbers	3 heads of romaine lettuce	1 head of iceberg lettuce
1 head of cauliflower	1 head of cabbage	2 heads of broccoli
1 big bunch of kale	1 big bunch or stalk of celery	1 small bunch of asparagus
fresh thyme, rosemary, and sage mixed	fresh basil leaves	fresh mint leaves
1 small bunch of coriander leaves	1 small bunch of parsley	1 small bunch of fresh dill
4 oz of fresh ginger root	3 limes	½ dozen lemons
½ pound of blueberries	1 pound of strawberries	½ pound of blackberries

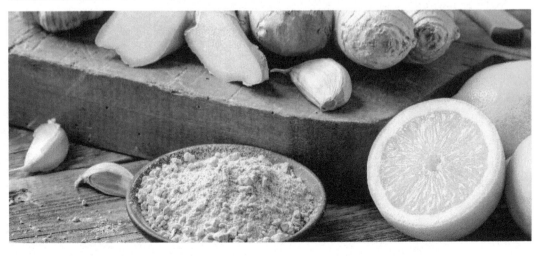

Proteins—Fresh or Frozen:

1.5 dozen eggs	½ pound of small shrimp	pack of bacon
1 pound of boneless chicken	1 whole chicken	

Dairy:

½ pound of unsalted butter	4 oz of Feta cheese	4 oz of cream cheese
4 oz of cheddar cheese	32 fl oz of almond milk	pint of heavy cream
8 oz of sour cream	1 pint of sugar-free vanilla ice cream	

Cooking Mediums:

16.9 fl oz of avocado oil	16.9 fl oz of coconut oil	16.9 fl oz of extra-virgin olive oil

Flours::

1 pound of super-fine almond flour

Condiments:

mayonnaise	peanut butter	yellow mustard
vanilla extract	peppermint extract	baking powder
16 fl oz of red wine vinegar	16 fl oz of apple cider vinegar	

Dried Herbs and Spices:

oregano	chili flakes	dried thyme, rosemary, and sage mixed
garlic powder	paprika powder	cumin powder
coriander powder	turmeric—ground	black pepper—ground
cinnamon	pumpkin pie spice	

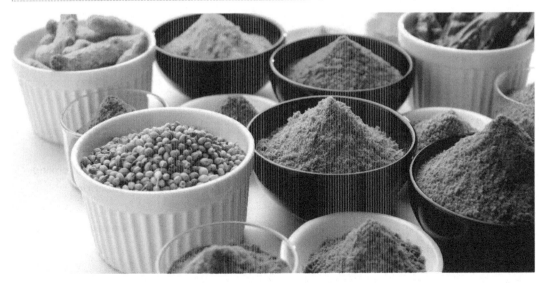

sliced black olives	sliced green olives	16.9 oz of grass-fed beef bone broth—pack of 2
8 fl oz of chicken broth—pack of 12	5 fl oz of vegetable broth—pack of 6	1 pound of pumpkin purée
1 pound of tomato purée	7 oz of konjac/shirataki noodles—pack of 4	Cauliflower rice

Snacks:

roasted salted pepitas	salted, roasted almonds	macadamia nuts
hazelnuts	dried black currants	Parmesan crisps

Week 2 Shopping List

Fresh Produce:

2 medium zucchini	2 cups of fresh baby spinach	garlic bulb
1-inch piece of fresh ginger	½ pound of plum tomatoes	½ pound of cherry tomatoes
2 onions (one white and one red)	1 pound of fresh green beans	3 cucumbers
1 head of romaine lettuce	1 head of iceberg lettuce	1 pound of small baking pumpkins
1 head of cabbage	2 heads of broccoli	1 small bunch of asparagus

fresh thyme, rosemary, and sage mixed	fresh basil leaves	fresh mint leaves
1 small bunch of coriander leaves	1 small bunch of parsley	1 small bunch of fresh dill
3 limes	4 lemons	½ pound of blueberries
pound of strawberries	½ pound of blackberries	

Proteins—Fresh or Frozen:		
1.5 dozen eggs	4 salmon fillets of 4 oz each—skin-on preferred	1 pound of boneless pork chops
1 pound of Italian sausage links	1 whole chicken	

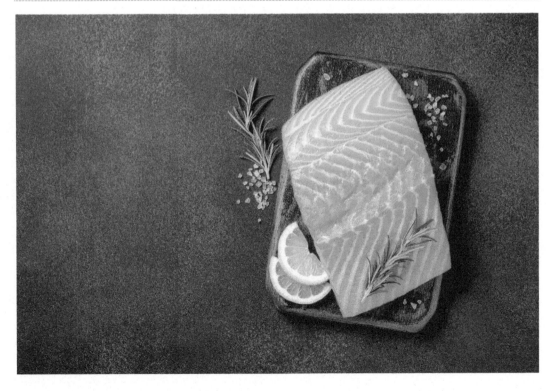

Dairy:

½ pound of unsalted butter	4 oz of Feta cheese	4 oz of cream cheese
4 oz of cheddar cheese	32 fl oz of almond milk	1 pint of heavy cream
8 oz of sour cream	16 oz pint of sugar-free vanilla ice cream	

Cooking Mediums:

16.9 fl oz of avocado oil	16.9 fl oz of coconut oil	16.9 fl oz of extra-virgin olive oil

Flours::

1 pound of coconut flour

Ready-To-Use:

sliced black olives	sliced green olives	16.9 oz of grass-fed beef bone broth—pack of 2
8 fl oz of chicken broth—pack of 12	5 fl oz of vegetable broth—pack of 6	7 oz of konjac/shirataki noodles—pack of 4
Cauliflower rice		Cauliflower rice

Snacks:

roasted, salted pepitas	salted, roasted almonds	macadamia nuts
hazelnuts	dried black currants	dried black currants

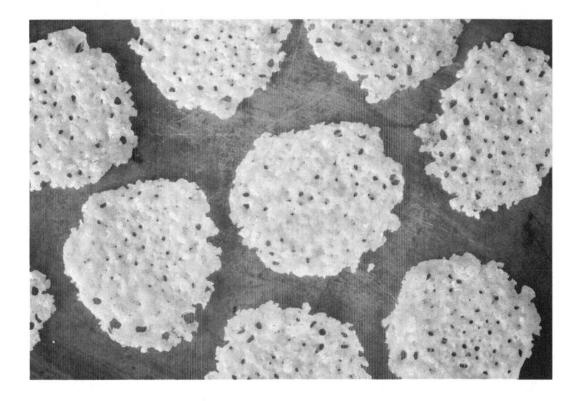

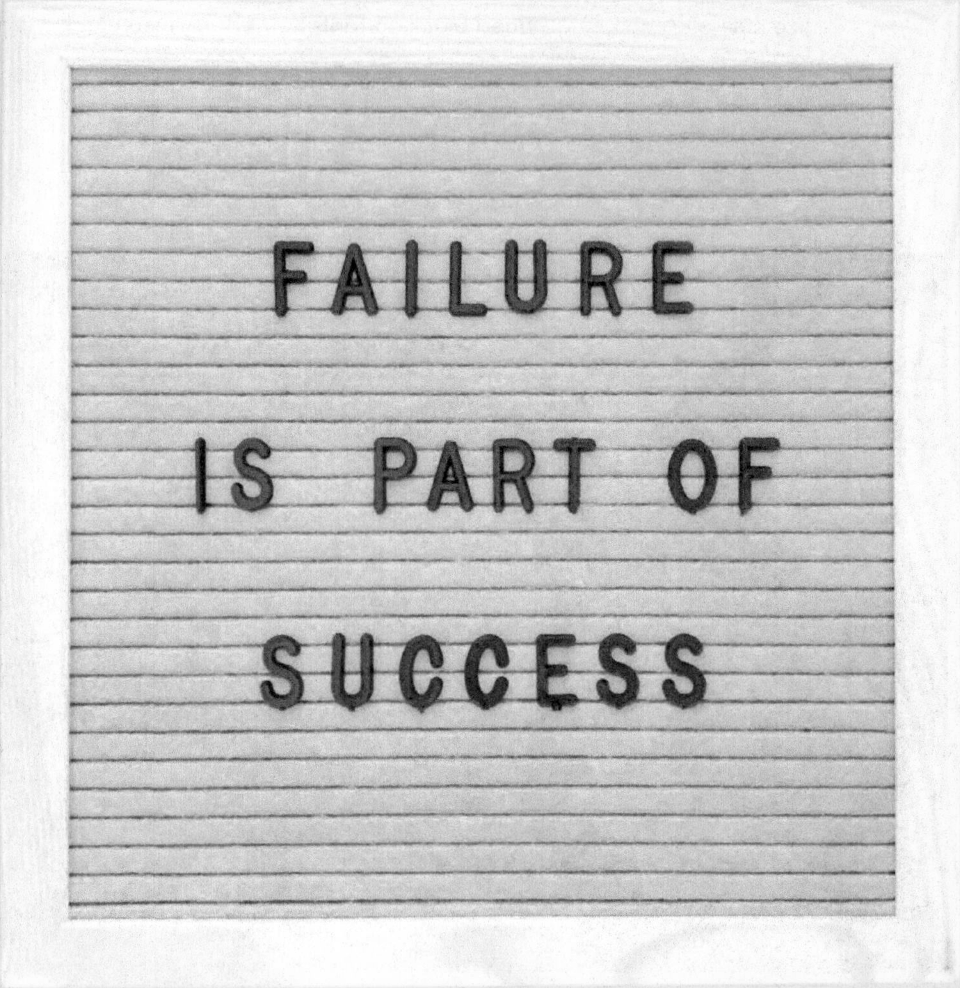
FAILURE
IS PART OF
SUCCESS

Chapter 16:
Neat-O Tips for Keto Success

Whether you are chasing weight loss or not, whether you follow keto or don't, you must not be hard on yourself—that is the most important tip for personal success. When you are having fun while doing whatever you are doing, everything feels perfectly fine.

Although, who doesn't like to bag some tips and tricks along the way? If you are really into something, getting a valuable tip from those who have been there and done that can be very helpful. To get the most out of anything in life, you need to learn the finer nitty-gritty details. Sometimes, you may come across a whole new take on the topic you want to gain mastery over; sometimes, even the old ways can have hidden gems for you.

Tips can act like those glow-in-the-dark markers along the streets that try to make the journey safer for you, and tricks could be like finding a hidden train platform that leads to Hogwarts. Tricks could be things that are open knowledge but are treated as trade secrets. Tricks can seem easy to the one who figures it out and yet a big puzzle to another. And for those who got the trick right, it can be pure magic; you could walk straight through the wall you have just hit, while facts are indeed hard and solid—those which you can base your decisions upon.

Let me see what kind of tips, tricks, and facts I can rustle up for you, so you can have some more fun while exploring your keto life and making way with fat loss.

Tips and Tricks

1. Go Easy on Your Meal Size

You do not have to think of three big meals a day. Rather, prepare for smaller meals and snacks spread over the eating window of your day. Ketosis is already suppressing your appetite. It is most likely that you won't finish that big meal like you used to before keto, so you do not need to fret about cooking up large meals. Think small, and go easy on your tummy.

2. Get Systematic about It

Have you played Jenga? Then you must know that the game is all about pulling one brick out at a time without toppling the tower. You think, plan, and strategize which food gets pulled out of your diet one after the other. Do not crash everything. Take the sugar sources out as a priority. The candies, carbonated drinks, and sugar in the beverages need to go out; followed by the processed foods such as pasta, bread, cakes and biscuits, rice, etc.; and then the starchy fruits and vegetables get pulled out.

3. Eat Different Fats

Fats are your friends, and you must not stick to just a few. The more different fats on your plate, the merrier your keto journey. So don't just include those saturated fats in your daily meal plan. Feel free to drizzle some extra-virgin olive oil over your seafood or cook in coconut oil. Too many fats from just meats and dairy are not advisable either.

4. Limit Those Proteins, Too

Most who start with keto often forget that protein is an important macro, too. Its ratio is as important as the other two especially because proteins in excess will supply amino acids to your body. By a process called gluconeogenesis, the acids get converted into sugar which can be detrimental to your keto weight loss strategy.

5. Drink Water for Better Weight Loss

Water not only keeps you from getting dehydrated during ketosis but also suppresses your appetite. Drinking water from time to time can keep you from feeling hungry. In the 1940s, the Food and Nutrition Board of the National Academy of Sciences recommended that adults drink 84 ounces of water per day. With time, this recommendation got transformed into the 8 x 8 rule which stipulates an intake of eight ounces of water eight times per day (Stanton, n.d.) yielding 64 ounces per day.

Sipping on berry-infused water can be beneficial for satisfying sugar cravings and hydrating your body at the same time.

6. Create Your Space

Not everyone in your family will want to eat as you do. Sometimes, unfortunately, families are not as supportive of the dietary changes that keto demands. In both cases, you should stock up your own pantry and keep some refrigerated items handy for keto cooking. Try to set aside space for yourself so you can store your ingredients, snacks, etc.

7. Think Out of the Box

Keto is an ingenious diet plan that was used in medicinal therapy then creatively applied for weight loss. Creating keto recipes to balance the macros also needs a bit of creativity. Since ketosis is already charging up your brain cells, you have nothing to lose. Expend some energy to think outside of the box and try making your own recipes from keto friendly ingredients in your pantry.

8. Join Keto Communities

Social media is a bonus in many ways. You can find keto communities on many platforms. Connecting with fellow keto dieters can be very useful. You can share tips and tricks that you learned from this book and get some new ones from your new keto circle. Birds of the keto feather can make a chirpy flock. Find yours! Join our new *Fun with Keto* Facebook group at www.facebook.com/groups/funwithketo and find your tribe.

9. Watch and Listen to Your Body

What are you following keto for? Your body. So learn to talk, listen, and watch your body. Yes, in front of the mirror would be a good place to start. Watch how your body is right now and keep noticing how it changes with time. Snap some full-length mirror selfies for the record. Measure your statistics with a tailor's sewing tape and note in a journal or use the MyFitnessPal app for that. Also, listen to what your body is telling you about the diet regimen and how it feels. Talk yourself into believing that you are going to make a success out of your keto mission. Then, cheer yourself on with a happy, "Yeeto!"

Fun Fact-O

This short and—dare I say—sweet list is not trivia. These are facts about keto that you must know. "Did you know?" is always an intriguing hook, especially when it comes to gossip, but we aren't wasting time here. These facts might bust some keto myths for you:

1. National Keto Day is celebrated on January 5th every year. Founded by The Vitamin Shoppe, the intention was to educate people about

the health benefits of the ketogenic diet and bring awareness about what the keto lifestyle offers.

2. While you are at it, you should also celebrate National Green Juice Day, National Nut Day, or National Better Breakfast Day and have some fun, memorable meals planned on the calendar. Mark the dates!

3. Intermittent fasting alone cannot lead to ketosis until after six or seven days. When the ketone levels in your body are anywhere between 1.5-6 mmol/L, you have entered the state of ketosis.

4. Ketone levels in any normal individual range between 0.6-1.5 mmol/L. A review published in 2017 in *The Journal of Physiology* said that the ketone levels in your blood after prolonged aerobic exercises reach a maximum of 2 mmol/L only, where extreme fasting for up to seven days elevated the blood ketone levels to qualify as nutritional ketosis (Keto, 2020).

5. Botanically bananas are berries, but a strawberry is not a berry at all: It consists of multiple fruits. Yet, for keto, bananas are off your pantry list, and strawberries are welcome.

6. After the emergence of drugs for epilepsy, the ketogenic diet waned in popularity and almost disappeared by the 1930s. It was only after the Meryl Streep-starring movie titled *First Do No Harm* was released in 1997 that it shot to fame once again. Charlie, the son of Jim Abrahams, the director of the movie, was treated for epilepsy with the help of the ketogenic diet at the Johns Hopkins Hospital. The Charlie Foundation for Ketogenic Therapies was founded in 1994 to provide information about diet therapies for people affected by epilepsy, other neurological disorders, and select cancers (The Charlie Foundation, n.d.-a).

Dieting effectively is what keto followers unanimously wish, and shedding that fat is a dream come true.

Here's one more success tip before we sign out:

> "Doing the best at this moment puts you in the best place for the next moment"
>
> **– Oprah Winfrey (Oprah Winfrey Quotes, n.d.).**

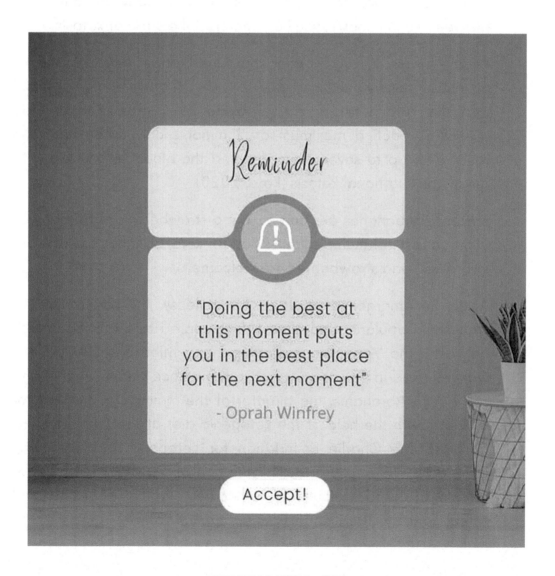

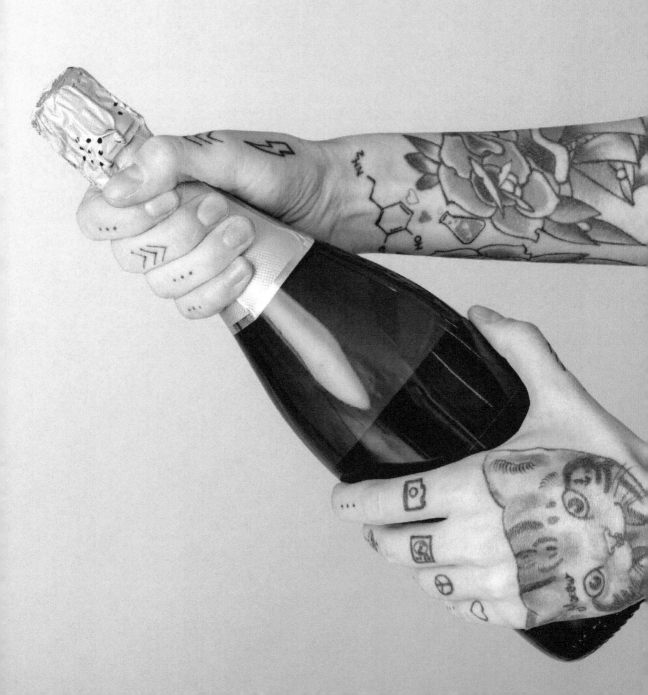

Conclusion

I selected a bottle of dry champagne off the rack and walked up to the checkout counter.

A big smile spread over the young lady's face as she scanned the Brut Champagne bottle for me.

"Celebrating something?" she asked good-naturedly as I handed over my credit card.

"Yeah! That there are only two grams of carbs, zero grams of fats, and zero grams of protein in every glass of this bubbly," I quipped.

Living with Yeeto

Make Yeeto a Morning Ritual

There's some kind of magic in the mornings. Take the energy of the rising sun and spread the sunshine liberally all over your day. It is a sweet treat but carb-free! *wink wink*

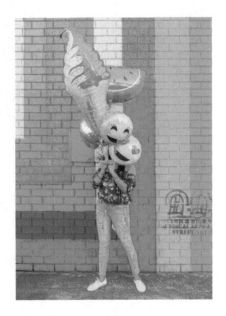

You are living the keto life from the minute your foot hits the ground. Drink a glass of warm water first. Your body needs it! Then, on to a bit of exercise maybe and a sip of a great cup of tea or coffee. Give a "Yeeto" and start your day.

I hope you will take this book along with you as you make daily progress in your weight-loss journey. Remember when you started with questions like, "Why is dieting so hard?" Yet everything changed when you realized that the simple answer is, "It wasn't fun." Then, finding a fun way of doing it feels nothing less than magic. I wish for you to successfully reduce your weight and elevate your life with the keto magic.

I hope you have developed a method of weaving the keto lifestyle into your daily routine. Planning your day from the previous night can keep things moving like a well-oiled machine—your regular life and keto life working together in a smooth tandem. It's counting your macros and picking some quick-prep keto meals, drinks, and snacks to keep you fueled through your day.

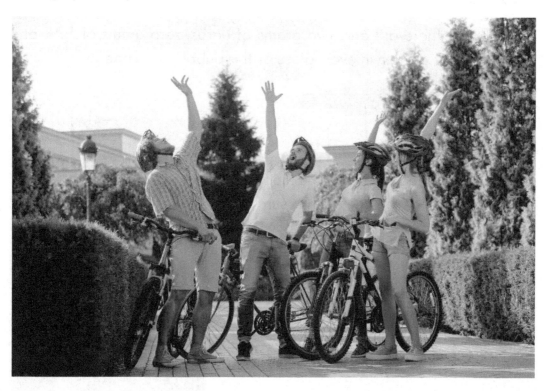

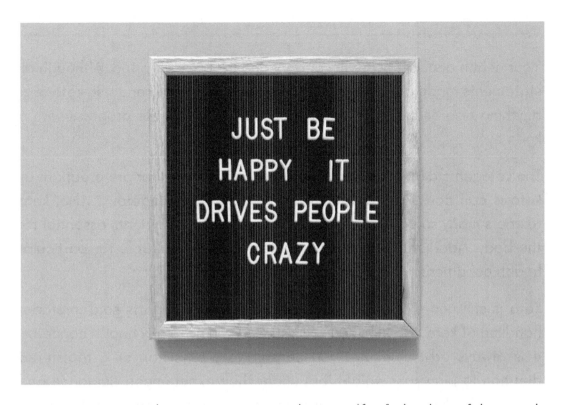

You can revisit Chapter 6 to remind yourself of the list of low-carb probiotics that you can include in your daily intake to improve your gut health. When you find your health improving along with substantial fat loss, don't forget you heard about the best supplement mix and the Garden of Life Grass-Fed Butter right here.

There are two days that you need to schedule out of your keto week or month according to your choice and convenience. The cheat day or the day you will have your cheat meal and one day to restock your pantry essentials. Based on Chapters 13 and 14, you have a two-week sample grocery list for your reference in Chapter 15.

Even if you hit a plateau with your weight loss, you do not need to worry. Chapter 10 is a champ; it is loaded with Yeeto hacks for keto success. Here's also hoping that the tips, tricks, and fun facts will help you continue on with keto and live with Yeeto!

Words of Caution

Your health and safety are my priority and responsibility, too. Although all statements made are scientifically-backed and I would endorse keto over anything else as a healthy lifestyle, you must track your progress with a keen eye.

The ketogenic diet is not for women trying to conceive or are pregnant as ketosis can cause dehydration which may prove dangerous. Also, keto restricts many sources of macronutrients and micronutrients essential for the body. Additionally, some supplements are not suitable for particular health conditions.

Keto is still under research in many areas. Some reports said improper handling of keto can trigger renal issues. If you have any health concerns, it is always advisable that you consult your physician or a registered dietitian to plan your weight loss under their experienced guidance and monitoring while following the intermittent fasting + ketogenic diet plan.

About The Authors:

Tony Scott and Stephen Rezza are just two regular guys who felt compelled to share their keto diet experience with the rest of the world. Their keto journey began as accountability partners to keep each other inspired and motivated to reach their weight-loss goals. The younger of the two, Stephen enjoys using the slang phrase "yeet" to celebrate his keto dieting achievements and discoveries. The two ultimately began affectionately referring to their diet as "YEETO" to maintain a spirit of excitement about shedding unwanted pounds and eating delicious keto-friendly foods. Tony is an author and marketing communications entrepreneur, and Stephen is an accomplished music artist and develops talent as A&R for BMGPM/Def7 Records. Both reside in Los Angeles, California.

References

Alothman, M., Hogan, S. A., Hennessy, D., Dillon, P., Kilcawley, K. N., O'Donovan, M., Tobin, J., Fenelon, M. A., & O'Callaghan, T. F. (2019). The "Grass-Fed" Milk Story: Understanding the Impact of Pasture Feeding on the Composition and Quality of Bovine Milk. *Foods, 8*(8), 350. https://doi.org/10.3390/foods8080350

art111111111. (2014). Bacon Salad. In *Pixabay*. https://pixabay.com/photos/bacon-salad-fresh-4515867/

Banse, L. (2018). Noodles. In *Unsplash*. https://unsplash.com/photos/FaUCROC_BZ8

Baum, I. (2020, July 7). *The Best Low-Carb Vegetables to Eat on Keto.* Men's Health. https://www.menshealth.com/nutrition/g26553021/best-keto-friendly-vegetables/

Bowers, E. S. (2014, October 6). *5 Essential Nutrients to Maximize Your Health.* EverydayHealth.com. https://www.everydayhealth.com/hs/guide-to-essential-nutrients/simple-guide-to-good-nutrition/

Bradley, S., & Santilli, M. (2020, August 28). *Tons of People Do Intermittent Fasting and Keto at the Same Time—But Is That a Good Idea?* Women's Health. https://www.womenshealthmag.com/weight-

https://cavemanketo.com/configuring-mfp/

The Charlie Foundation. (n.d.-a). *About Us*. Charlie Foundation. https://charliefoundation.org/about-us/

The Charlie Foundation. (n.d.-b). *Studies on the Ketogenic Diet for Brain Health*. Charlie Foundation. https://charliefoundation.org/am-i-a-candidate/keto-for-brain-health/

DoctorNDTV. (2019, June 12). *5 Keto-Friendly Probiotics to Prevent Digestion Problems during Summer*. NDTV.com. https://www.ndtv.com/health/5-keto-friendly-probiotics-to-prevent-digestion-problems-during-summer-2049659

Erdman, J., Oria, M., & Pillsbury, L. (2011). *Nutrition and Traumatic Brain Injury: Improving Acute and Subacute Health Outcomes in Military Personnel*. Nih.gov; National Academies Press (US). https://www.ncbi.nlm.nih.gov/books/NBK209323/

Escape, N. (2016). Infused Water. In *Pixabay*. https://pixabay.com/photos/infused-water-water-juice-1830178/

Fraust, A. (2020). Cauliflower Rice. In *Unsplash*. https://unsplash.com/photos/VswX66fwP3Q

Gaffney, Y. (2020). Vegetable Salad. In *Unsplash*. https://unsplash.com/photos/V1K5Z5KERsw

Garza, J. M. (2019). *Keto-Friendly Recipes: Easy Keto for Busy People*. Houghton Mifflin Harcourt.

Gavin, M. L. (2018, June). *Easy Exercises for Teens*. Kidshealth.org. https://kidshealth.org/en/teens/easy-exercises.html

Grabkowska, M. (n.d.). Bowl of Pumpkin Soup. In *Unsplash*.

https://unsplash.com/photos/w-R_sfcakP0

Gunnars, K. (2020, April 20). *Intermittent Fasting 101—The Ultimate Beginner's Guide*. Healthline. https://www.healthline.com/nutrition/intermittent-fasting-guide#effects

Hamzic, H. (2018, November 9). *Keto Macros: A Guide to Understanding Nutrient Ratios*. Kiss My Keto Blog. https://blog.kissmyketo.com/articles/keto-diet-basics/keto-macros-a-guide-to-understanding-nutrient-ratios/

Haney, A. (2020). Eating. In *Unsplash*. https://unsplash.com/photos/CAhjZmVk5H4

Healthguru. (2017). Keto. In *Pixabay*. https://pixabay.com/photos/keto-diet-nutritious-snack-vitamin-5534051/

Hedonic treadmill. (2019, February 19). In *Wikipedia*. https://en.wikipedia.org/wiki/Hedonic_treadmill

Holiday, J. (2017). Salmon Pasta. In *Pixabay*. https://pixabay.com/photos/salmon-salmon-fillet-skin-food-2283787/

Holland, K. (2019, August 16). *Keto Diet May Help Fight Certain Cancers*. Healthline. https://www.healthline.com/health-news/what-to-know-about-keto-diet-and-cancer#A-new-focus-for-cancer-treatment

Johns Hopkins Medicine. (2021). *Intermittent Fasting: What Is It, and How Does It Work?* HopkinsMedicine.org. https://www.hopkinsmedicine.org/health/wellness-and-prevention/intermittent-fasting-what-is-it-and-how-does-it-work

Johns Hopkins Medicine. (n.d.). *Your Digestive System: 5 Ways to Support Gut*

Health. HopkinsMedicine.org.
https://www.hopkinsmedicine.org/health/wellness-and-prevention/your-digestive-system-5-ways-to-support-gut-health

Keto. (2020, September 26). *25 Secret Facts about Ketogenic Diet (Fun Facts).* YouTube.
https://www.youtube.com/watch?v=tfLAGZMWjNY&t=1s

Keto Products | Garden of Life. (n.d.). Garden of Life. Retrieved September 24, 2021, from https://www.gardenoflife.com/keto

KetoVale, T. (2019, May 10). *9 Best Probiotic Foods for Low Carb and Keto Diet.* KetoVale. https://www.ketovale.com/probiotic-foods/

Khazan, O. (2016, April 20). *How "Cheat Days" Help You Lose Weight.* The Atlantic. https://www.theatlantic.com/health/archive/2016/04/its-my-cheat-day/478881/

Kim, J.-M. (2017). Ketogenic Diet: Old Treatment, New Beginning. *Clinical Neurophysiology Practice, 2,* 161–162.
https://doi.org/10.1016/j.cnp.2017.07.001

Kim, K.-H., Kim, Y. H., Son, J. E., Lee, J. H., Kim, S., Choe, M. S., Moon, J. H., Zhong, J., Fu, K., Lenglin, F., Yoo, J.-A., Bilan, P. J., Klip, A., Nagy, A., Kim, J.-R., Park, J. G., Hussein, S. M., Doh, K.-O., Hui, C., & Sung, H.-K. (2017). Intermittent Fasting Promotes Adipose Thermogenesis and Metabolic Homeostasis via VEGF-Mediated Alternative Activation of Macrophage. *Cell Research, 27*(11), 1309–1326.
https://doi.org/10.1038/cr.2017.126

Laustkehlet. (2021). Mushroom Soup. In *Pixabay.*
https://pixabay.com/photos/mushroom-soup-mushroom-soup-dinner-6134689/

Lawler, M. (2020, April 16). *10 Types of the Keto Diet and How They Work*. EverydayHealth.com. https://www.everydayhealth.com/ketogenic-diet/diet/types-targeted-keto-high-protein-keto-keto-cycling-more/

Leonard, J. (2020, January 17). *16:8 Intermittent Fasting: Benefits, How-To, and Tips*. Medical News Today. https://www.medicalnewstoday.com/articles/327398#health-benefits

Lindberg, S. (2018, August 23). *Autophagy: Definition, Diet, Fasting, Cancer, Benefits, and More*. Healthline. https://www.healthline.com/health/autophagy#diet

Masood, W., & Uppaluri, K. R. (2019, March 21). *Ketogenic Diet*. Nih.gov; StatPearls Publishing. https://www.ncbi.nlm.nih.gov/books/NBK499830/

McKinney, D. (n.d.). Health and Wellness. In *Unsplash*. https://unsplash.com/photos/__QqvTI5Edc

Meixner, M. (2019, May 28). *7 Health Benefits of Grass-Fed Butter*. Healthline. https://www.healthline.com/nutrition/grass-fed-butter#TOC_TITLE_HDR_2

Migala, J. (2019, January 29). *Intermittent Fasting Keto: How It Works, Benefits, Risks, More*. EverydayHealth.com. https://www.everydayhealth.com/ketogenic-diet/intermittent-fasting-keto-how-it-works-benefits-risks-more/

Milkshake, C. (2020). Milkshake. In *Unsplash*. https://unsplash.com/photos/uttpvPp-Zlo

Miller, J. (2014). "Do You Bant?" William Banting and Bantingism: A Cultural History of a Victorian Anti-Fat Aesthetic. *English Theses & Dissertations*. https://doi.org/10.25777/xda4-7y41

Mossholder, T. (2018). Eat. In *Unsplash*.
https://unsplash.com/photos/FH3nWjvia-U

Mullens, A. (2021, June 17). *How to Break a Keto Weight Loss Stall*. Diet Doctor.
https://www.dietdoctor.com/weight-loss/break-a-stall

MyFitnessPal. (2016, March 21). *MyFitnessPal Restaurant Logging: Now on iOS
and Android*. MyFitnessPal Blog.
https://blog.myfitnesspal.com/myfitnesspal-introduces-restaurant-
logging/

Nada, L. (2018). Happy Face. In *Unsplash*.
https://unsplash.com/photos/tXz6g8JYYoI

Nut, A. (2010). Shrimps Salad. In *Pixabay*.
https://pixabay.com/photos/shrimps-salad-food-healthy-fresh-
646677/

Oprah Winfrey Quotes. (n.d.). BrainyQuote. Retrieved September 29, 2021,
from https://www.brainyquote.com/quotes/oprah_winfrey_121212

Oxford Dictionary. (n.d.). *YEET*. Lexico Dictionaries | English.
https://www.lexico.com/definition/yeet

Paoli, A., Bosco, G., Camporesi, E. M., & Mangar, D. (2015). Ketosis, Ketogenic
Diet and Food Intake Control: A Complex Relationship. *Frontiers in
Psychology*, *6*. https://doi.org/10.3389/fpsyg.2015.00027

Paoli, A., Mancin, L., Bianco, A., Thomas, E., Mota, J. F., & Piccini, F. (2019).
Ketogenic Diet and Microbiota: Friends or Enemies? *Genes*, *10*(7), 534.
https://doi.org/10.3390/genes10070534

quotespedia.org. (n.d.). *Confucius*. Quotespedia. Retrieved September 13,
2021, from https://www.quotespedia.org/authors/c/confucius/it-

does-not-matter-how-slowly-you-go-as-long-as-you-do-not-stop-
confucius/

Ramos, A. (2016). *Complete Ketogenic Diet for Beginners: Your Essential
Guide to Living the Keto Lifestyle*. Callisto Media.

RitaE. (2017). Pancakes. In *Pixabay*. https://pixabay.com/photos/pancakes-
schaumomelette-omelette-1984693/

Robinson, L., Segal, R., & Smith, M. (October 2020). *Best Exercises for Health
and Weight Loss*. Help Guide.
https://www.helpguide.org/articles/healthy-living/what-are-the-best-
exercises-for-me.htm

Rose, E. (2018, April 25). *Apple Cider Vinegar's Benefits: Lose Weight, Heal
Your Gut and Treat Acne*. Bulletproof.
https://www.bulletproof.com/supplements/dietary-
supplements/apple-cider-vinegar-benefits/

Rose, J. (2020). Chicken Soup. In *Unsplash*.
https://unsplash.com/photos/1hzdlacVPyl

Saunion, S. (2019, November 19). *Here's How to Properly Calculate Your Keto
Macros*. Eat This Not That. https://www.eatthis.com/keto-macros-
calculator/

Sifferlin, A. (2017, May 25). The Weight Loss Trap: Why Your Diet Isn't Working.
TIME, 189(21). https://time.com/magazine/us/4793878/june-5th-2017-
vol-189-no-21-u-s/

Spritzler, F. (2021, June 18). *Can Keto or Low-Carb Diets Improve Acne?* Diet
Doctor. https://www.dietdoctor.com/low-carb/benefits/acne

Stanton, B. (n.d.). *How Much Water Do You Need on Keto?* Carb Manager.

https://www.carbmanager.com/article/xtqwcbeaaceacgke/how-much-water-should-i-drink-on-keto/

StockSnap. (2016). Green Smoothie. In *Pixabay*. https://pixabay.com/photos/green-smoothie-strawberries-fruit-2607334/

Szalay, J. (2015, December 10). *What Is Protein?* Live Science. https://www.livescience.com/53044-protein.html

Tentis, D. (2017). Shakshuka. In *Plxabay*. https://pixabay.com/photos/kagyana-strapatsada-gdarta-2955104/

Urban Dictionary: Yeet. (2019). Urban Dictionary. https://www.urbandictionary.com/define.php?term=Yeet

Wellversed Health. (2020, August 20). *Why Is Salt Needed in the Keto Diet?* Wellversed. https://wellversed.in/blogs/articles/why-is-salt-needed-in-the-keto-diet

Zuzyusa. (2018). Ketodieta. In *Pixabay*. https://pixabay.com/photos/food-diet-keto-ketodieta-fitness-3223286/

Made in the USA
Coppell, TX
16 July 2022

79879685R00109